Aids to Anatomy

To our long suffering wives
Sheila and Ruth

Aids to Anatomy

Simon Paterson-Brown
MB BS FRCS(Ed) FRCS
Research Fellow and Honorary Surgical Registrar,
Academic Surgical Unit,
St Mary's Hospital Medical School, London

Rupert Eckersley
MB BS FRCS
Research Fellow and Honorary Surgical Registrar,
Academic Surgical Unit,
St Mary's Hospital Medical School, London

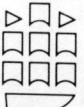

CHURCHILL LIVINGSTONE
EDINBURGH LONDON MELBOURNE AND NEW YORK 1988

CHURCHILL LIVINGSTONE
Medical Division of Longman Group UK Limited

Distributed in the United States of America by Churchill Livingstone Inc., 1560 Broadway, New York, N.Y. 10036, and by associated companies, branches and representatives throughout the world.

© Longman Group UK Limited 1988

All rights reserved. No part of this publication may be reproduced, stored in a retrieval system, or transmitted in any form or by any means, electronic, mechanical, photocopying, recording or otherwise, without the prior permission of the publishers (Churchill Livingstone, Robert Stevenson House, 1–3 Baxter's Place, Leith Walk, Edinburgh EH1 3AF).

First published 1988

ISBN 0-443-03624-1

British Library Cataloguing in Publication Data
Paterson-Brown, Simon
  Aids to anatomy.
  1. Anatomy, human
  I. Title II. Eckersley, Rupert
  611   QM23.2

Library of Congress Cataloging in Publication Data
Paterson-Brown, Simon.
  Aids to anatomy.

  1. Anatomy, Human—Handbooks, manuals, etc.
  2. Anatomy, Surgical and topographical—Handbooks, manuals, etc. I. Eckersley, Rupert. II. Title.
  [DNLM: 1. Anatomy—handbooks. QS 39 P296o]
  QM23.2.P29 1988   611'.0076   87-25016

Produced by Longman Singapore Publishers (Pte) Ltd.
Printed in Singapore.

Preface

Having sat both undergraduate and postgraduate anatomy examinations within the last few years it became apparent to us how useful a short book made up of anatomical notes and lists would be for revision purposes. This book is the result of our thoughts, notes and impressions which we have collected together from our experiences in undergraduate second MB and postgraduate surgical anatomy examinations. A book of this size cannot hope to encompass all of anatomy. We hope, however, if used in conjunction with a standard anatomy textbook and a basic knowledge of the subject, that it will be helpful in revision for undergraduate exams, as well as for the postgraduate exams which involve the detailed anatomical knowledge as required for the primary FRCS and radiology examinations.

This book has been structured according to 'systems' with a view to easy reference and the information has been taken from Gray's anatomy.

We are grateful for the help and guidance we have received from Churchill Livingstone and we are indebted to Angela Samuel for her tolerance and expertise in producing the manuscript.

London, S. P-B
1988 R. E.

Contents

Cardiovascular system	1
Lymphatic system, spleen and thymus	30
Nervous system	39
Respiratory system	68
Gastrointestinal system	76
Genito-urinary system	105
Peritoneum	123
Myology	127
Arthrology	172
Osteology	175
Orbit, ear and nose	191
Fossae, triangles and canals	203
Endocrine glands	213
Skin and breast	220

Cardiovascular system

HEART
The heart is a four-chambered muscular organ occupying the middle mediastinum. It lies behind the sternum, anterior to the oesophagus and pulmonary veins and between the two pleural cavities. Inferiorly it is attached to the conjoint tendon of the diaphragm by the fibrous pericardium, which fuses superiorly with the great vessels.

PERICARDIUM

Layers
The pericardium surrounds the heart and consists of two layers:
1. Fibrous: external layer
2. Serous
   a. parietal
   b. visceral
   The two serous layers form the oblique and transverse sinuses

Nerve supply
Phrenic nerve

Blood supply
1. Pericardiacophrenic artery
2. Internal thoracic artery
3. Branches of thoracic aorta

Venous drainage
To azygos system of veins

STRUCTURE

Macroscopic
There is a fibrous skeleton around which the cardiac muscle of the heart is attached. This consists of fibrous rings surrounding each atrioventricular orifice and the pulmonary and aortic orifices. The Bundle of His is the only structure which crosses this fibrous skeleton.

Atrial fibres
1. Superficial: common to both atria
2. Deep: separate to each atria

Ventricular fibres
A complex arrangement of superficial and deep fibres which are common to both ventricles and form the papillary muscle of each ventricle.

Microscopic
Each muscle cell is elongated and has a centrally placed nucleus. It may partially divide at its end to connect to other muscle cells by intercalated discs. Cardiac muscle resembles a network of branching and anastomosing cylinders.

CHAMBERS

There are particular features for each chamber.

Right atrium (RA)
1. Auricle
2. Sulcus terminalis
3. Musculi pectinati
4. Coronary sinus: posterior and below the superior vena cava opening
5. Inferior vena cava opening
6. Tricuspid valve: leading to right ventricle
7. Fossa ovalis: extending up to annulus ovalis
8. Interatrial septum: posteromedial wall
9. Superior vena cava opening

Right ventricle (RV)
1. Trabeculae carnae: muscular ridges, one of which forms the moderator band
2. Tricuspid valve (three cusps)
   a. anterior
   b. inferior
   c. septal
3. Papillary muscle: with chordae tendineae
4. Pulmonary orifice (three cusps)
   a. posterior
   b. anterior (two)
5. Interventricular septum
6. Infundibulum

Left atrium (LA)
1. Auricle
2. Four pulmonary orifices

3. Mitral valve: leading to left ventricle (LV)
4. Musculi pectinati

Left ventricle (LV)
1. Trabeculae carneae: no moderator band
2. Papillary muscle: with chordae tendineae
3. Mitral valve (two cusps)
   a. anterior
   b. inferior
4. Aortic vestibule
5. Interventricular septum
   a. membraneous part
   b. muscular part
   (the pars membranacea forms the membraneous upper part of the interventricular septum)
6. Aortic valve (three cusps)
   a. anterior
   b. posterior (two)

ARTERIAL SUPPLY

Right coronary artery
Supplies:
1. Anterior wall of RA
2. Lower part of RA
3. Inter-atrial septum
4. Most of RV
5. Small strip of LV
6. Interventricular septum
7. Sinu-atrial node (55%)
8. Atrioventricular node
9. Bundle of His

Left coronary artery
Supplies:
1. Upper margin of RV
2. Most of LV
3. Interventricular septum
4. Posterior wall of RA
5. Left and right auricular appendages
6. Lower part of LA
7. Inter-atrial septum
8. Sinu-atrial node (45%)
9. Atrioventricular node (occasionally)
10. Bundle of His

VENOUS DRAINAGE

The following veins drain the heart:
1. Great cardiac vein
2. Left marginal vein
3. Posterior vein of left ventricle
4. Middle cardiac vein
5. Small cardiac vein
6. Oblique vein of left atrium (of Marshall)
7. Anterior cardiac veins
8. Venae cordis minimae

NERVE SUPPLY

Vagus nerve

Cardio-inhibitor
1. Superior cardiac branch
2. Inferior cardiac branch

Sympathetic nerve supply

Cardio-accelerator from superficial and deep cardiac plexuses
Supplied by:
1. Superior cervical ganglion
2. Middle cervical ganglion } on each side
3. Inferior cervical ganglion

Conducting system

This is made up of specially differentiated muscle, namely nodal and purkinge fibres.

Sinu-atrial node (SAN)
This lies on the upper part of the sulcus terminalis of the right atrium, extending medially in front of the opening of the superior vena cava. Impulses are transmitted by muscle fibres from SAN to the atrioventricular node (AVN).

Atrioventricular node (AVN)
This lies above the opening of the coronary sinus into the right atrium, in the atrial septum.

Atrioventricular Bundle of His
This runs from the AVN through the pars membranaceae, divides into right and left branches and is distributed to the ventricular muscle by subendocardial plexuses of Purkinge fibres.

DEVELOPMENT

The heart develops from a single heart tube. This elongates, bends and rotates to form the mature heart.

Endocardial cushions grow in to separate atrial and ventricular cavities, and the septae divide the atria and ventricles into right and left.

The heart tube is made up of five parts:
1. Sinus venosus: forms the atria
2. ＿＿＿＿＿＿＿＿＿ : part of the sinus venosus forms the coronary sinus
3. Atria: forms the atria
4. Ventricle: forms the ventricles
5. Truncus arteriosus: forms the aortic and pulmonary trunk

SYSTEMIC ARTERIAL SYSTEM

The systemic arterial system originates from the left ventricle as the aorta.

AORTA

The branches of the aorta are as follows.

Ascending aorta
1. Right coronary artery
2. Left coronary artery

Arch of aorta
Brachiocephalic trunk which in turn gives rise to:
1. Right common carotid artery
2. Right subclavian artery
3. Thyroidea ima artery
4. Thymic artery
5. Left common carotid artery
6. Left subclavian artery

Descending thoracic aorta
1. Pericardial arteries
2. Bronchial arteries: one on right, two on left
3. Oesophageal arteries: four to five branches
4. Mediastinal arteries
5. Phrenic arteries
6. Posterior intercostal arteries
    a. dorsal branches: spinal and muscular
    b. collateral
    c. muscular

d. lateral cutaneous
   e. mammary: second to fourth spaces
   f. right bronchial artery

Abdominal aorta
1. Inferior phrenic arteries (right and left)
2. Coeliac trunk
3. Middle suprarenal arteries (right and left)
   a. renal branches
   b. inferior suprarenal branch
4. Superior mesenteric artery
5. Renal arteries (right and left)
6. Gonadal arteries (right and left)
7. Inferior mesenteric artery
8. Lumbar arteries
9. Median sacral artery

Termination of aorta
Common iliac arteries (right and left)

CORONARY ARTERIES

Right coronary artery
Four main branches:
1. Marginal branch
2. Posterior interventricular branch
3. Branch to atrioventricular node
4. Branch to sinu-atrial node (55%)

Left coronary artery
Three main branches:
1. Anterior interventricular branch
2. Circumflex artery: continuation of left coronary artery
3. Branch to sinu-atrial node

COMMON CAROTID ARTERY

The right and left common carotid arteries usually have no branches and bifurcate at the level of the 3rd and 4th cervical vertebrae into right and left internal and external carotid arteries. The branches of both right and left sides are the same.

Internal carotid artery
1. Caroticotympanic artery
2. Pterygoid branch (in the Pterygoid canal)
3. Cavernous branch
4. Hypophysial branch
5. Meningeal branch
6. Ophthalmic artery

Cardiovascular system 7

   a. central artery of retina
   b. posterior ciliary artery
   c. lacrimal artery
   d. anterior ciliary artery: to muscles of orbit
   e. medial palpebral artery
   f. ethmoidal artery
      (i) anterior
      (ii) posterior
   g. supra-orbital artery ⎫ These branches anastomose with
   h. supratrochlear artery ⎬ branches of the maxillary, facial
   i. dorsal nasal artery ⎭ and superficial temporal arteries
7. Anterior cerebral artery (right and left): joined by anterior communicating artery
8. Middle cerebral artery
9. Posterior communicating artery
10. Choroidal artery

External carotid artery
1. Superior thyroid artery
   a. superior laryngeal artery
   b. infrahyoid artery
   c. cricothyroid artery
2. Ascending pharyngeal artery
   a. pharyngeal artery
   b. inferior tympanic artery
   c. meningeal artery
3. Lingual artery
   a. suprahyoid artery
   b. dorsal lingual artery
   c. sublingual artery
   d. ends as arteria profunda linguae
4. Facial artery
   a. ascending palatine artery
   b. tonsillar artery
   c. submental artery
   d. labial artery
   e. facial branches
   f. angular artery: termination of facial artery
   g. glandular branches
5. Occipital artery
   a. muscular branches
   b. mastoid branches
   c. descending branch
      (i) superficial
      (ii) deep
   d. meningeal branch
   e. occipital branch
6. Posterior auricular artery

8   Aids to anatomy

    a. stylomastoid artery
    b. auricular branch
    c. occipital branch
7. Superficial temporal artery
    a. transverse facial artery
    b. anterior auricular artery
    c. zygomatico-orbital artery
    d. middle temporal artery
       (i) frontal branch
       (ii) parietal branch
8. Maxillary artery: divided into three parts
    1st part
    a. middle meningeal artery
    b. accessory meningeal artery
    c. deep auricular artery
    d. inferior alveolar artery
    e. anterior tympanic artery
    2nd part
    a. muscular branches
       (i) pterygoids ($\times 2$)
       (ii) temporalis
       (iii) masseter
       (iv) buccal
    3rd part
    a. posterior superior alveolar artery
    b. infra-orbital artery
    c. greater (anterior) palatine artery
    d. sphenopalatine artery
    e. pharyngeal branch

The branches of the third part of the maxillary artery accompany the branches of the pterygopalatine ganglion.

SUBCLAVIAN ARTERY

The right and left subclavian arteries are divided into three by the scalenus anterior muscle. The branches from both sides are the same except where indicated.

First part
Four major branches:
1. Vertebral artery
    a. muscular branches
    b. spinal branches
    c. meningeal branches
    d. medullary branches
    e. posterior inferior cerebellar artery
    f. posterior spinal artery
    g. anterior spinal artery

This terminates by joining the opposite side forming the *basilar artery* which gives the following branches:
- a. pontine branches
- b. anterior inferior cerebellar arteries (right and left)
- c. labyrinth arteries: several on each side
- d. superior cerebellar arteries (right and left)
- e. posterior cerebral artery, this communicates with the internal carotid artery through the posterior communicating artery

2. Internal mammary artery
   - a. anterior intercostal arteries
   - b. pericardiacophrenic artery
   - c. mediastinal branches
   - d. perforating (to skin) branches
   - e. musculophrenic artery
   - f. superior epigastric artery
3. Thyrocervical trunk
   - a. inferior thyroid artery
     - (i) ascending cervical artery
     - (ii) inferior laryngeal artery
     - (iii) tracheal branches
     - (iv) oesophageal branches
     - (v) terminal to thyroid gland
   - b. superficial cervical artery
   - c. suprascapular artery
4. Left costocervical trunk
   - a. superior intercostal artery
   - b. deep cervical artery
   - c. dorsal scapular artery

Second part
Right costocervical trunk

Third part
This usually has no branches, but occasionally gives off the dorsal scapular artery.
Termination: continues as the *axillary artery* at the outer border of the 1st rib.

The transverse cervical artery (when present) comes off the thyrocervical trunk and divides into:
1. Superficial cervical artery
2. Dorsal scapular artery

Scapular anastomosis
Formed from branches of:
1. Suprascapular artery
2. Subscapular artery
3. Deep branch of transverse cervical artery

AXILLARY ARTERY

The right and left axillary arteries are divided into three parts of pectoralis minor muscle.

First part
Superior thoracic artery

Second part
1. Acromiothoracic artery
   a. pectoral branch
   b. acromial branch
   c. clavicular branch
   d. deltoid branch
2. Lateral thoracic artery: gives lateral mammary branches in the female

Third part
1. Subscapular artery
   a. circumflex scapular artery
   b. infrascapular artery
2. Anterior circumflex humeral artery
3. Posterior circumflex humeral artery

Termination: becomes the brachial artery at the lower border of teres major.

BRACHIAL ARTERY

1. Profunda brachii artery
   a. nutrient branch
   b. deltoid branch
   c. middle collateral branch*
   d. radial collateral branch*
   e. other muscular branches
2. Main nutrient artery: to humerus
3. Superior ulnar collateral artery*: accompanies ulnar nerve
4. Inferior ulnar collateral artery*
5. Muscular branches: to coracobrachialis, biceps and brachialis muscles
6. *Radial Artery*
7. *Ulnar Artery*

* These arteries are involved in the anastomosis around the elbow joint.

RADIAL ARTERY

1. Radial recurrent artery: involved in elbow joint anastomosis
2. Muscular branches: to muscles on radial side of forearm
3. Palmar carpal branch
4. Superficial palmar branch
5. Dorsal carpal branch
6. First dorsal metacarpal artery
7. Arteria princeps pollicis ⎫ these may start in common as
8. Arteria radialis indicis ⎭ the 1st palmar metacarpal artery

ULNAR ARTERY

1. Anterior ulnar recurrent artery
2. Posterior ulnar recurrent artery
3. Common interosseous artery: muscular branches
    a. anterior interosseous artery: nutrient branches (to ulna and radius) : median artery (accompanies the median nerve
    b. posterior interosseous artery: the interosseous recurrent artery and is involved with elbow joint anastomosis)
4. Muscular branches
    a. palmar carpal branch
    b. dorsal carpal branch
    c. deep palmar branch

CARPOPALMAR ARCHES

These arches give branches which supply the bones and muscles of the wrist and hand.

Deep palmar arch
Formed from
1. Terminal part of radial artery
2. Deep palmar branch of ulnar artery

It lies over the proximal ends of the metacarpal bones.

Branches
1. Three palmar metacarpal arteries: run distally on the interosseous muscles of the metacarpal spaces. They join the common digital branches of the superficial palmar arch
2. Three perforating branches: pass through the 2nd, 3rd and 4th interosseous spaces to anastomose with the dorsal metacarpal arteries
3. Recurrent branches: supply carpal bones, ending in the palmar carpal arch

Superficial palmar arch
This is formed from the ulnar artery and the superficial palmar branch of the radial artery.

Branches
Three common palmar digital arteries pass distally along the 2nd, 3rd and 4th lumbricals. They are joined by the palmar metacarpal arteries of the deep palmar arch, and then divide into a pair of palmar digital arteries. These run distally along the sides of the index, middle, ring and little fingers, dorsal to the corresponding digital nerves. Each digital artery gives off two dorsal branches.

Dorsal carpal arch
This is formed from the dorsal carpal branch of the ulnar and radial arteries.
   It forms three dorsal metacarpal arteries which bifurcate to form the dorsal digital arteries.

Palmar carpal arch
This is formed from palmar carpal branch of ulnar and radial arteries. It supplies the wrist and carpus.

COELIAC TRUNK

This is a short, wide vessel, which comes off the front of the aorta at the level of the 12th thoracic vertebrae (T12) just below the aortic hiatus in the diaphragm.
It has three branches:
1. Left gastric artery
2. Hepatic artery
3. Splenic artery

Left gastric artery

Branches
1. Lower oesophagus
2. Cardia of stomach
3. Lesser curvature of stomach down to pylorus: anastomoses with branches of splenic artery and right gastric artery

Hepatic artery

Branches
1. Right gastric artery
   a. pylorus
   b. lesser curve of stomach (anastomosing with left gastric artery)
   c. it may give supraduodenal artery
2. Gastroduodenal artery
   a. right gastroepiploic artery
   b. superior pancreaticoduodenal artery
3. Right hepatic artery
4. Left hepatic artery

The cystic artery can be a branch of the right or left hepatic artery or even the main hepatic artery.

Anatomical variations of the hepatic artery
1. The hepatic artery may arise from the superior mesenteric artery or the aorta
2. An accessory left hepatic artery may arise from the left gastric artery
3. An accessory right hepatic artery may arise from the superior mesenteric artery

Splenic artery
1. Pancreatic branches: one of which is arteria pancreatica magna
2. Short gastric arteries (vasa brevia)
3. Left gastroepiploic artery
4. Five terminal branches to spleen

SUPERIOR MESENTERIC ARTERY

The superior mesenteric artery (SMA) supplies the small intestine from below the superior part of the duodenum to the caecum, the ascending and most of the transverse colon. It originates from the front of the aorta about 1 cm below the coeliac trunk at the level of the first lumbar vertebrae (L1). After passing anterior to the uncinate process of the pancreas and crossing the horizontal part of the duodenum it enters the root of the mesentery.

Branches
1. Inferior pancreaticoduodenal artery
   a. anterior branch ⎫ anastomose with corresponding branches
   b. posterior branch ⎭ of superior pancreaticoduodenal artery
2. Jejunal and ileal branches 12–15 from left side of SMA. These form a series of arches with each other within the mesentery of the small intestine.
3. Ileocolic artery (from right of SMA)
   a. superior branch: anastomoses with right colic artery
   b. inferior branch
      (i) ascending (colic) branch
      (ii) anterior ⎫ caecal branches
      (iii) posterior ⎭
      (iv) appendicular artery
      (v) ileal branch: anastomoses with termination of SMA
4. Right colic artery (from the right side of the middle of SMA)
   a. ascending branch: anastomoses with middle colic artery at hepatic flexure
   b. descending branch: anastomoses with ileocolic artery

5. Middle colic artery leaves the SMA just below the pancreas
   a. right branch: anastomoses with right colic artery
   b. left branch: anastomoses with left colic artery

Other branches: occasionally the SMA may give origin to:
1. The common hepatic artery
2. The gastroduodenal artery
3. An accessory right hepatic artery

GONADAL ARTERIES

The right and left gonadal arteries come off the front of the aorta just below the renal arteries, which come off the aorta at the level of the second lumbar vertebrae (L2).

Right and left gonadal arteries

Branches
1. Perirenal fat
2. Ureter
3. Iliac lymph nodes
4. Cremaster and testis
5. Ovary: a branch continues to the uterus along the fallopian tube, anastomoses with uterine artery and then runs in round ligament to labia majora through canal of Nuck

INFERIOR MESENTERIC ARTERY

The inferior mesenteric artery (IMA) comes off the front of the aorta at the level of the 3rd lumbar vertebrae (L3) behind the horizontal part of the duodenum. It supplies the left third of the transverse colon, the descending colon, sigmoid colon and rectum.

Branches
1. Left colic artery
   a. ascending branch (anastomoses with middle colic artery)
   b. descending branch (anastomoses with highest sigmoid artery)
2. Sigmoid arteries
   Two or three in number, they supply the sigmoid colon and anastomose with left colic artery superiorly and the superior rectal artery inferiorly
3. Superior rectal artery
   This is the continuation of the IMA into the pelvis after it has given off its sigmoid branches. It divides opposite the 3rd sacral vertebrae (S3) into two branches which supply the rectum.

These branches communicate with:
1. Middle rectal artery: branch of the internal iliac artery
2. Inferior rectal artery: branch of the internal pudendal artery

Cardiovascular system 15

COMMON ILIAC ARTERIES
The abdominal aorta bifurcates at the lower level of the 4th lumbar vertebrae (L4). The right and left common iliac arteries divide into external and internal iliac arteries over the sacro-iliac joints on each side. Both common iliac arteries may give branches to:
1. Peritoneum
2. Ureter
3. Psoas Major

Internal iliac artery
It divides into anterior and posterior trunks at upper margin of the greater sciatic foramen. Branches are the same for both right and left.

Branches from anterior trunk
1. Superior vesical artery
    a. bladder
    b. ureter
    c. ductus deferens
2. Inferior vesical artery
    a. bladder
    b. ureter
    c. prostate
    d. seminal vesicles
3. Vaginal artery
    a. vagina
    b. bladder
    c. bulb of vestibule
4. Middle rectal artery
    a. rectal muscle
    b. seminal vesicles
    c. prostate
5. Uterine artery
    a. ureter
    b. cervix uteri
    c. vagina
    d. uterus
    e. uterine tube: anastomoses with ovarian artery
    f. round ligament
6. Obturator artery
    a. inside pelvis
        (i) iliac ⎫
        (ii) vesical ⎬ branches
        (iii) pubic ⎭
    b. outside pelvis
        (i) anterior branch: muscle
        (ii) posterior branch: muscles and acetabular branch

An abnormal obturator artery may be a branch of the inferior epigastric artery.
7. Internal pudendal artery
    a. muscles of pelvis
    b. perineal branches
    c. artery of bulb (of penis or vestibular bulb in female)
    d. inferior rectal artery
    e. urethral artery
    f. deep artery of penis/clitoris (supplies erectile tissue of corpus cavernosum)
    g. dorsal artery of penis/clitoris
8. Inferior gluteal artery
    a. muscular branches
    b. artery to sciatic nerve
    c. descending anastomotic branch to cruciate anastomosis on femur
    d. articular branch to hip
    e. cutaneous branches

Branches from the posterior trunk
1. Iliolumbar artery
    a. lumbar
    b. spinal } branches
    c. iliac
2. Lateral sacral arteries: superior and inferior branches
3. Superior gluteal artery: divides into superficial and deep branches after leaving the pelvis through the greater sciatic foramen above piriformis
    Branches of superior gluteal artery
    Within pelvis to
        a. piriformis
        b. obturator internus
        c. innominate bone
    Outside pelvis
        a. superficial branch
        b. deep branch   } to gluteal muscle

External iliac artery
Branches on both sides are the same
1. Inferior epigastric artery
    a. cremasteric artery
    b. pubic artery
    c. abdominal muscles
    d. anastomoses with superior epigastric artery
2. Deep circumflex iliac artery: to anterior superior iliac spine
Termination: the external iliac artery becomes the femoral artery as it enters the thigh under the inguinal ligament.

Femoral artery
1. Superficial epigastric artery
2. Superficial circumflex iliac artery
3. Superficial external pudendal artery
4. Deep external pudendal artery
5. Muscular branches
6. Profunda femoris artery: arises from lateral side of femoral artery, 3–4 cm below inguinal ligament

Branches of profunda femoris
1. Lateral circumflex femoral
    a. ascending branch
    b. descending branch
    c. transverse branch
2. Medial circumflex femoral
    a. ascending branch
    b. transverse branch
    c. acetabular branch
3. Muscular branches: numerous
4. Descending genicular artery
5. Perforating arteries: usually three
6. The profunda artery terminates as the 4th perforating artery

Cruciate anastomosis
This lies on the femur below the insertion of quadriceps femoris at the level of the lesser trochanter. It is formed from:
1. Descending branch of the inferior gluteal artery
2. Ascending branch of the 1st perforating artery
3. Transverse branch of the lateral circumflex femoral artery
4. Transverse branch of the medial circumflex femoral artery

Termination: the femoral artery becomes the popliteal artery after it passes through the hiatus in adductor magnus.

Popliteal artery
The popliteal artery traverses the popliteal fossa, dividing at the lower border of popliteus into anterior and posterior tibial arteries.

Branches
1. Cutaneous
2. Muscular
3. Genicular
    a. superior genicular
        (i) medial
        (ii) lateral
    b. middle genicular
    c. inferior genicular
        (i) medial
        (ii) lateral

4. Anterior tibial artery: descends anterior to the interosseous membrane, terminating as the dorsalis pedis artery on the dorsum of the foot

Branches of anterior tibial artery:
1. Posterior tibial recurrent artery
2. Anterior tibial recurrent artery
3. Muscular branches (numerous)
4. Anterior medial malleolar artery
5. Anterior lateral malleolar artery
6. Arteries around ankle joint
7. Dorsalis pedis artery
8. Lateral tarsal artery
9. Medial tarsal artery
10. Arcuate artery
    a. 2nd ⎫
    b. 3rd ⎬ dorsal metatarsal arteries
    c. 4th ⎭
5. Posterior tibial artery
    a. circumflex fibular artery
    b. peroneal artery
       (i) muscular
       (ii) nutrient to fibula
       (iii) anastomosing at ankle joint
    c. nutrient: to tibia
    d. muscular
    e. medial malleolar branches
    f. Calcanean branches

Terminates: as the medial plantar artery and the lateral plantar artery to form the plantar arch.

Plantar arch

Branches of the plantar arch
1. Perforating arteries (×3)
2. Plantar metatarsal arteries: each divides into two digital arteries

SYSTEMIC VENOUS SYSTEM

The right atrium receives blood from three main sources:
1. Superior vena cava
2. Inferior vena cava
3. Coronary veins

SUPERIOR VENA CAVA

Formed from: left and right brachiocephalic veins

Receives: azygos vein

Right Brachiocephalic vein

Formed from:
1. Right internal jugular vein
2. Right subclavian vein

Receives:
1. Right vertebral vein
2. Right internal thoracic vein
3. Right inferior thyroid vein: drains
   a. thyroid gland
   b. trachea
   c. oesophagus
   d. inferior laryngeal vein
4. Right first posterior intercostal vein (supreme)

Left brachiocephalic vein

Formed from:
1. Left internal jugular vein
2. Left subclavian vein

Receives:
1. Left vertebral vein
2. Left internal thoracic vein
3. Left inferior thyroid vein
4. Left superior intercostal vein (receives 2nd, 3rd and 4th posterior intercostal veins)
5. Left 1st posterior intercostal vein (supreme)
6. Thymic veins
7. Pericardial veins

Azygos vein
The azygos vein ascends from its origin as the lumbar azygos vein below the diaphragm through the posterior mediastinum on the right of the front of the bodies of the thoracic vertebrae. It arches forward at the level of the fourth thoracic vertebrae to end in the superior vena cava. It receives the posterior intercostal veins and the bronchial veins on the right side.

The hemi-azygos and the accessory hemi-azygos veins form the equivalent venous channel on the left side. Both communicate with the azygos vein, and also each other. The lumbar azygos vein is formed from the right ascending lumbar vein and the right subcostal vein.

Internal jugular vein
Formed from the sigmoid sinus as it enters the jugular foramen. The tributaries on the right and left side are the same.

Tributaries
1. Inferior petrosal sinus
2. Pharyngeal veins
3. Common facial vein
   a. anterior facial vein
   b. anterior branch of retromandibular vein
4. Lingual vein
5. Occipital vein: may join the posterior auricular vein
6. Superior thyroid vein
   a. thyroid gland
   b. superior laryngeal vein
   c. cricothyroid vein
7. Middle thyroid vein
   a. thyroid gland
   b. larynx
   c. trachea

It is worth noting the venous drainage of the face, as there are important extracranial-intracranial communications which can result in the spread of infection from the face into the cranial cavity. (See Fig. 1)

Cranial venous sinuses

The cranial sinuses form a venous network between the two layers of the dura mater. They drain blood from the brain (via cerebral veins) and bones of the cranium (via diploic veins). Most of them drain into the sigmoid sinus which becomes the internal jugular vein as it enters the jugular foramen (see Fig. 2).

It is important to note the communication between intra- and extracranial veins (via emissary veins) because inflammatory processes outside the skull may travel inwards through emmissary veins, leading to thrombosis in the sinuses, a serious and often fatal condition.

Intracranial	*Extracranial*
Cavernous sinus	Pterygoid plexus (via foramen ovalis)
	Pharyngeal veins (via foramen lacerum)
Middle meningeal vein	Pterygoid plexus
Ophthalmic veins	Anterior facial vein
Sigmoid sinus	Suboccipital plexus
	Posterior auricular vein (via mastoid emissary vein)
Occipital sinus	Internal vertebral plexus (via foramen magnum)
Superior saggital sinus	Nasal veins (via foramen caecum if patent)
	Scalp veins (via parietal emissary vein)

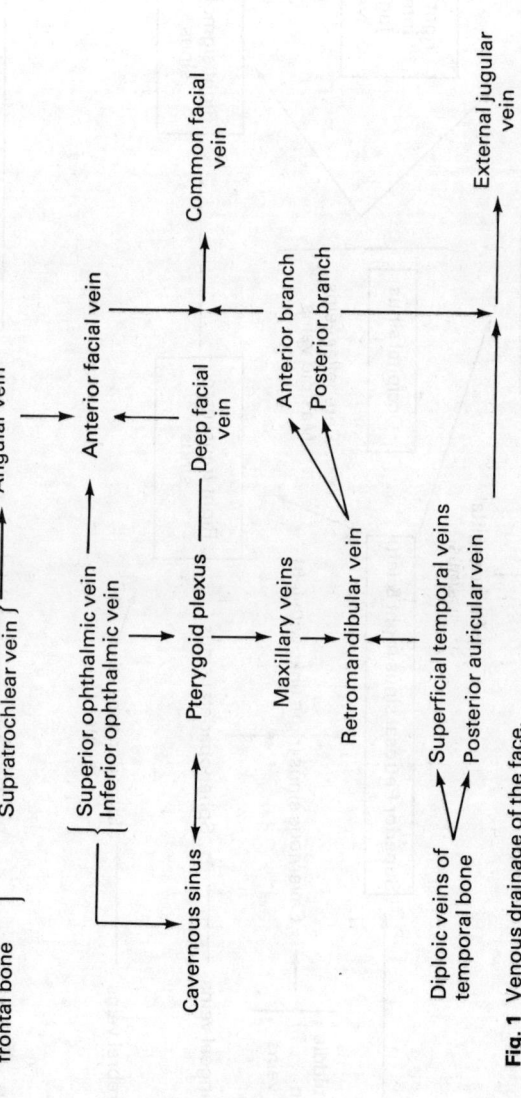

Fig. 1 Venous drainage of the face.

22 Aids to anatomy

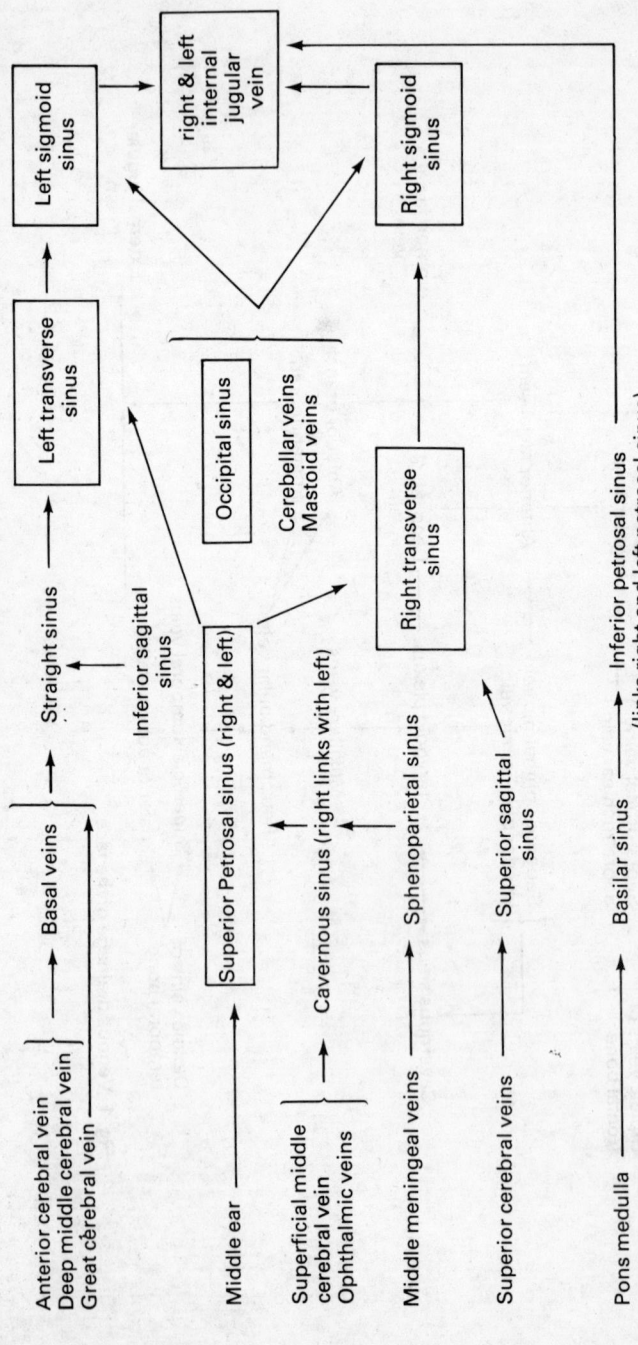

Fig. 2 Drainage of cranial venous sinuses.

Subclavian vein

This is the continuation of the axillary vein as it crosses the outer border of the 1st rib. It joins the internal jugular vein at the medial border of scalenus anterior forming the brachiocephalic vein.

Tributaries
1. External jugular vein
2. Dorsal scapular vein
3. Anterior jugular vein
4. Thoracic duct into left subclavian vein
5. Right lymphatic duct into right subclavian vein

Axillary vein

The axillary vein is the continuation of the basilic vein at the lower border of teres major.

Tributaries
1. Brachial veins ($\times 2$) (at lower end of subscapularis)
2. Cephalic vein (below clavicle)
3. Other tributaries correspond to the branches of the axillary artery

Venous drainage of the upper limb
1. Superficial veins
   dorsal venous arch drains to:
   a. median central vein
   b. cephalic vein (lateral side)
   c. basilic vein (medial side) which becomes axillary vein
2. Deep veins

These accompany the ulnar and radial arteries becoming the brachial veins on each side of the brachial artery.

INFERIOR VENA CAVA

The inferior vena cava (IVC) drains the lower limbs, abdomen and pelvis. It is formed from the right and left common iliac veins on the right of the 5th lumbar vertebrae.

It passes behind the right common iliac artery to ascend on the right of the abdominal aorta. It is contained within a groove in the liver and perforates the central tendon of the diaphragm at the level of the 8th thoracic vertebrae to the right of the midline behind the 6th costal cartilage, to enter the right atrium of the heart.

Tributaries
1. Hepatic veins
   a. right
   b. left
   c. middle

2. Right inferior phrenic vein
3. Left inferior phrenic vein
4. Right suprarenal vein
5. Left renal vein: passes in front of aorta
   a. left inferior phrenic vein
   b. left suprarenal vein
   c. left kidney
   d. left gonadal vein
6. Right renal vein
7. Right gonadal vein
8. Lumbar veins (×4)
   a. muscle and skin of loins
   b. abdominal wall
   c. vertebral plexuses
   The lumbar veins are connected by the ascending lumbar vein

Common iliac vein
Formed from external and internal iliac veins which join to form the common iliac vein in front of the sacroiliac joint.

Tributaries (on each side)
1. Iliolumbar vein
2. Lateral sacral veins
3. Median sacral vein: drains into left common iliac vein

Internal iliac vein
Drains:
1. Gluteal veins (superior and inferior)
2. Internal pudendal vein
   Receives:
   a. prostate and venous plexus of:
      (i) bladder
      (ii) prostate
   b. deep dorsal vein of penis
   c. scrotum/labia
   d. bulb of penis
3. Obturator vein
4. Lateral sacral veins
5. Middle rectal veins
   Receives:
   from inferior rectal veins and external rectal venous plexus, but communicates with the superior rectal vein via the internal rectal venous plexus.
6. Vesical veins
   a. bladder
   b. prostate
   c. seminal vesicles
   d. vesical venous plexus

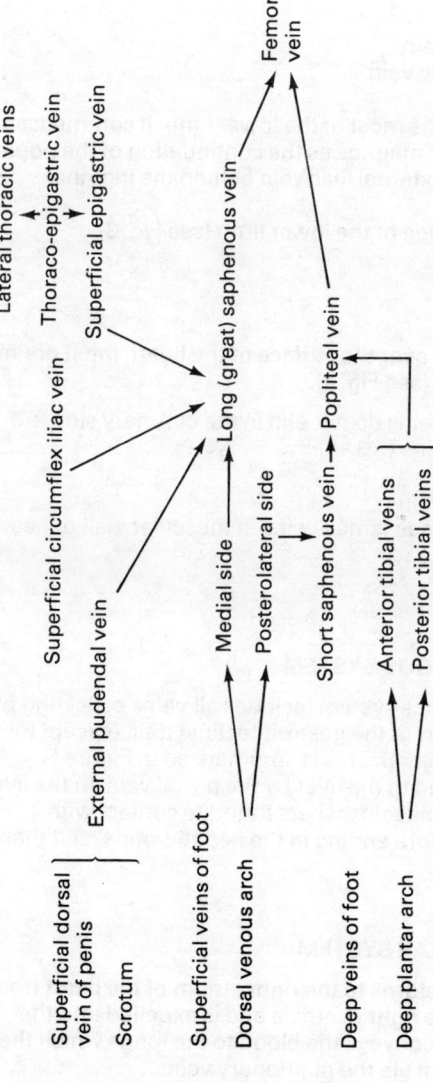

Fig. 3 Venous drainage of the lower limb. Note the thoraco-epigastric vein provides a link between the areas of venous drainage of the superior and inferior vena cava.

External iliac vein
This vein is the upward continuation of the femoral vein as it passes behind the inguinal ligament.

Tributaries
1. Inferior epigastric vein
2. Deep circumflex iliac vein
3. Pubic vein

The femoral vein drains most of the lower limb. It commences at the opening in adductor magnus as the continuation of the popliteal vein and becomes the external iliac vein behind the inguinal ligament.

For the venous drainage of the lower limb (see Fig. 3).

CORONARY VEINS

The coronary veins run over the surface of the heart, most draining into the coronary sinus (see Fig. 4).

The following cardiac veins do not end in the coronary sinus:
1. Anterior cardiac veins (×3–4)
   a. right atrium
   b. right marginal vein
2. Venae cordis minimae (small veins in muscular wall of heart)
   a. atria
   b. ventricles

HEPATIC PORTAL VENOUS SYSTEM

The hepatic portal venous system includes all veins collecting blood from the abdominal part of the gastrointestinal tract (except for the lower part of the anal canal). This is summarized in Figure 5.

The blood is conveyed to the liver by the portal vein. In the liver this vein divides into sinusoids where intimate contact with hepatocytes occurs before ending in the hepatic veins, and then to the inferior vena cava.

PULMONARY VASCULAR SYSTEM

Deoxygenated blood returns to the right atrium of the heart from where it passes into the right ventricle and is expelled into the pulmonary trunk. This conveys the blood to the lungs which then returns to the left atrium via the pulmonary veins.

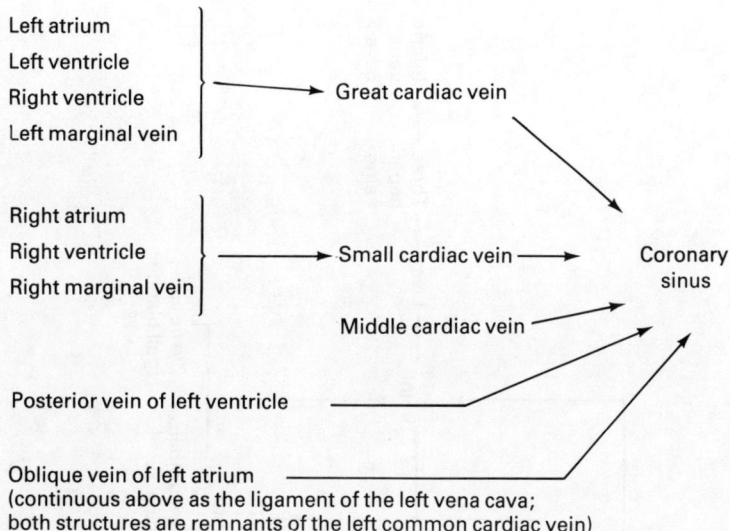

Fig. 4 Drainage of coronary veins.

PULMONARY ARTERIAL SUPPLY

The pulmonary trunk is 5 mm in length and 3 mm in diameter. It divides in the concavity of the aorta (at the level of the 5th thoracic vertebrae) into the right and left pulmonary arteries.

Right pulmonary artery

Superior branch
1. Upper lobe
   a. apical
   b. anterior descending
   c. anterior ascending
   d. posterior descending
   e. posterior ascending

Inferior branch
1. Middle lobe
   a. lateral branches
   b. medial branches
2. Lower lobe
   a. superior
   b. subsuperior
   c. medial basal
   d. anterior basal

28 Aids to anatomy

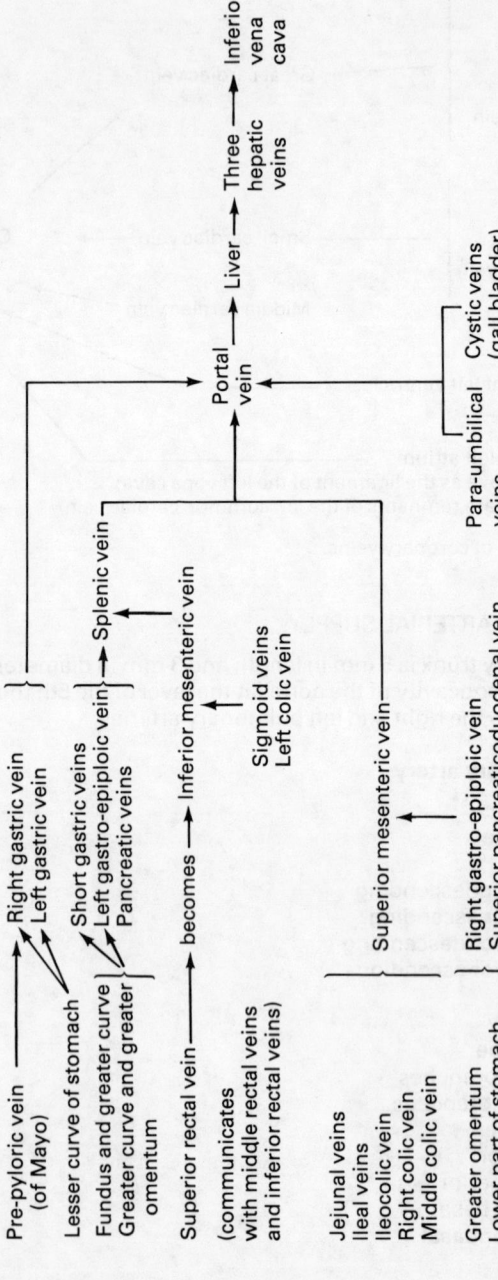

Fig. 5 Hepatic portal venous system.

e. lateral basal
  f. posterior basal

Left pulmonary artery

Upper branch
1. Apical
2. Posterior
3. Anterior descending
4. Anterior ascending
5. Lingular branch

Lower branch
1. Superior
2. Subsuperior
3. Medial basal
4. Anterior basal
5. Posterior basal

PULMONARY VENOUS SYSTEM

The pulmonary capillaries form plexuses in the walls of the alveoli and air saccules. They coalesce into larger branches, running through the substance of the lung independently to the arteries and bronchi. They ultimately form larger veins which come into relation with the arteries and bronchi. For the *pulmonary venous drainage*, see Figure 6.

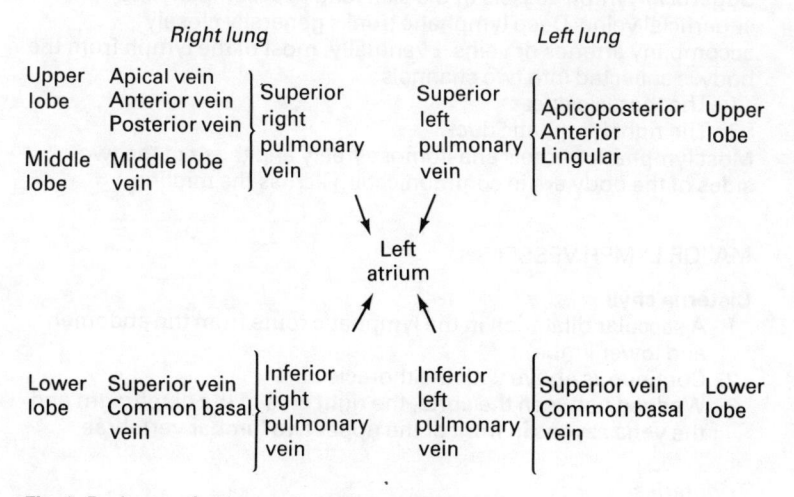

	Right lung			Left lung	
Upper lobe	Apical vein Anterior vein Posterior vein	Superior right pulmonary vein	Superior left pulmonary vein	Apicoposterior Anterior Lingular	Upper lobe
Middle lobe	Middle lobe vein				
		↘	↙		
		Left atrium			
		↗	↖		
Lower lobe	Superior vein Common basal vein	Inferior right pulmonary vein	Inferior left pulmonary vein	Superior vein Common basal vein	Lower lobe

Fig. 6 Drainage of pulmonary venous system.

Lymphatic system, spleen and thymus

LYMPHATIC SYSTEM

About 10–20% of tissue fluid formed at the arterial end of the capillary bed traverses the lymphatic system before returning to the venous system. In addition to transporting and modifying lymph, parts of the lymphatic system are involved in phagocytosis, altering immune responses and contributing to the cell population of the blood and lymph.

The lymphatic system comprises:
1. Lymph capillaries: commence in tissue spaces and empty lymph into certain veins
2. Lymph nodes: small solid masses of lymphoid tissue
3. Epitheliolymphoid tissue: collections of lymphoid tissue in the gastrointestinal tract, spleen and thymus
4. Circulating lymphocytes

Superficial lymph vessels of the skin tend to accompany the superficial veins. Deep lymphatic trunks generally closely accompany arteries or veins. Eventually, most of the lymph from the body is collected into two channels:
1. The thoracic duct
2. The right lymphatic duct

Most lymphatic vessels anastomose freely and those of the two sides of the body are in communication across the midline.

MAJOR LYMPH VESSELS

Cisterna chyli
1. A saccular dilatation in the lymphatic route from the abdomen and lower limbs
2. Continuous above with the thoracic duct
3. Wedged between the aorta, the right crus of the diaphragm and the vena azygos in front of the upper two lumbar vertebrae

Tributaries
1. Right and left lumbar trunks
2. Intestinal trunks

Thoracic duct
1. The common trunk of all lymph vessels of the body except those drained by the right lymphatic duct
2. About 38–45 cm long in the adult
3. Begins at the upper end of the cisterna chyli
4. Enters the thorax through the aortic opening
5. Ascends through the posterior mediastinum with aorta on its left and azygos vein on its right
6. Opposite T5, it inclines to the left and ascends to the thoracic inlet along the left of the oesophagus
7. In the neck, it arches laterally at the level of C7 transverse process
8. Runs anterior to the vertebral artery and vein, sympathetic trunk and thyrocervical trunk and branches
9. Passes in front of the phrenic nerve and medial border of scalenus anterior separated by prevertebral fascia
10. Passes behind the left common carotid artery, vagus nerve and internal jugular vein
11. Descends in front of the first part of the left subclavian artery
12. Ends by opening into the junction of the left subclavian and internal jugular veins

Tributaries
1. Abdomen: descending trunk from lower six or seven intercostal spaces on each side
2. Thorax
   a. lumbar trunk draining the upper lumbar lymph nodes on each side
   b. efferents from posterior mediastinal nodes
   c. intercostal lymph efferents from upper six left intercostal spaces
3. Neck
   a. left jugular trunk and left subclavian trunk may join the thoracic duct
   b. sometimes the left bronchomediastinal trunk

Right lymphatic duct
1. About 1 cm in length
2. Courses along the medial border of scalenus anterior
3. Ends by opening into the junction of the right subclavian and internal jugular veins

Tributaries
1. Right jugular trunk: from right half of head and neck
2. Right subclavian trunk: from right upper limb
3. Right bronchomediastinal trunk: from right thorax, lung, heart, convex surface of liver

These tributaries may join the right brachiocephalic vein separately.

MAJOR PATHWAYS OF LYMPHATIC DRAINAGE

```
                                              Left jugular trunk
                                              Left arm
                                              Posterior half of left thorax
                                                    |
                                                    v
Left brachiocephalic vein <-- Left subclavian vein <-- Thoracic duct <-- Cysterna chyli <-- Right and left lumbar trunks <-- Para-aortic nodes <-- Common iliac nodes
                                                                              ^
                                                                              |
                                                                        Pre-aortic nodes <-- Intestine

                    Bronchomediastinal trunk
                    Internal thoracic trunk
                    Right arm
                         |
                         v
Right brachiocephalic vein <-- Right jugular trunk
                         ^
                         |
                  Right lymphatic duct
                         ^
                         |
                  Posterior half of right thorax
```

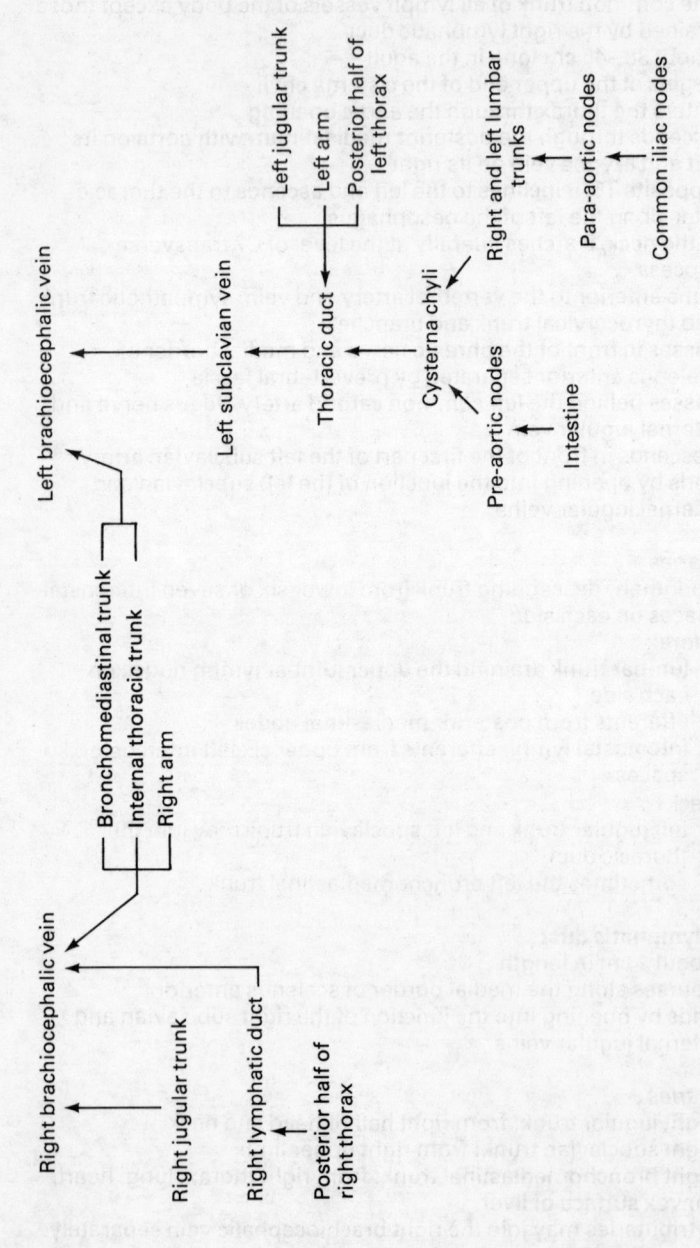

Fig. 7 The major pathways of lymphatic drainage.

REGIONAL LYMPHATIC DRAINAGE
Lower limb and pelvis

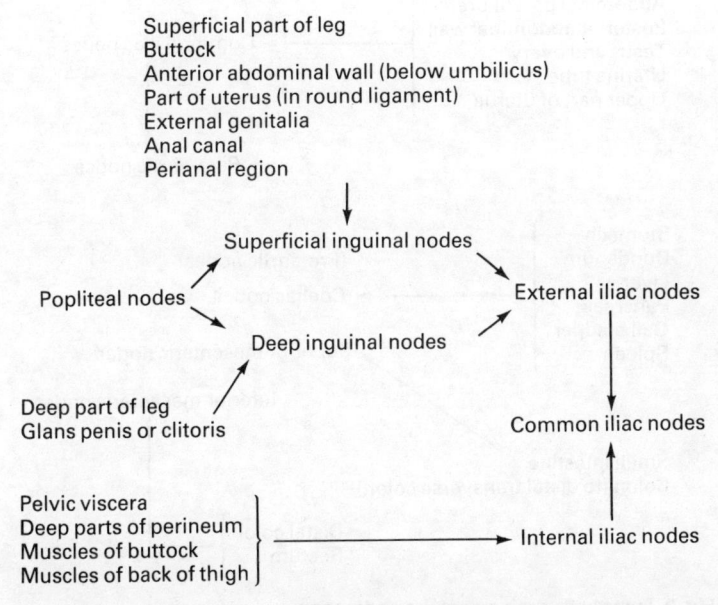

Superficial part of leg
Buttock
Anterior abdominal wall (below umbilicus)
Part of uterus (in round ligament)
External genitalia
Anal canal
Perianal region

↓

Popliteal nodes → Superficial inguinal nodes → External iliac nodes
       ↘ Deep inguinal nodes ↗
                ↓
Common iliac nodes
                ↑
Deep part of leg
Glans penis or clitoris → Deep inguinal nodes

Pelvic viscera
Deep parts of perineum
Muscles of buttock
Muscles of back of thigh → Internal iliac nodes

Fig. 8 Lymphatic drainage of the lower limb and pelvis.

Abdomen

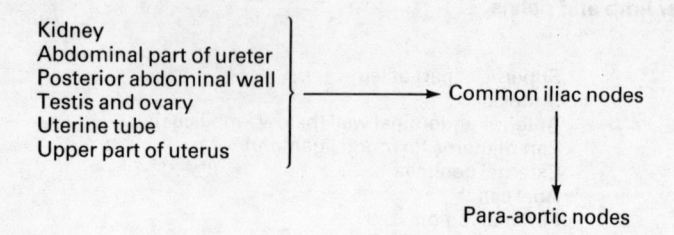

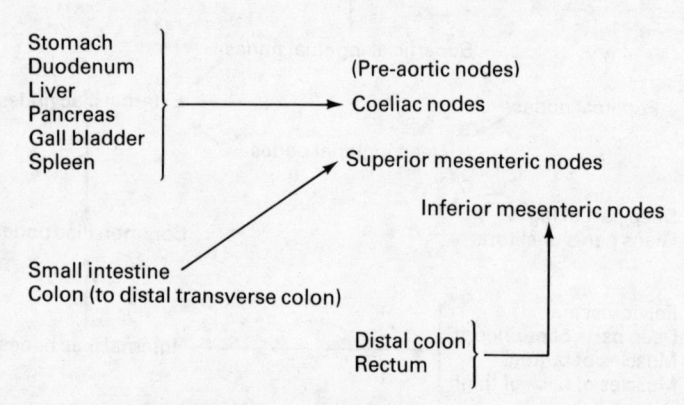

Kidney
Abdominal part of ureter
Posterior abdominal wall
Testis and ovary
Uterine tube
Upper part of uterus
} → Common iliac nodes → Para-aortic nodes

Stomach
Duodenum
Liver
Pancreas
Gall bladder
Spleen
} → (Pre-aortic nodes) Coeliac nodes

Small intestine
Colon (to distal transverse colon)
→ Superior mesenteric nodes

Distal colon
Rectum
} → Inferior mesenteric nodes

Fig. 9 Lymphatic drainage of the abdomen.

Upper limb

Axillary lymph nodes

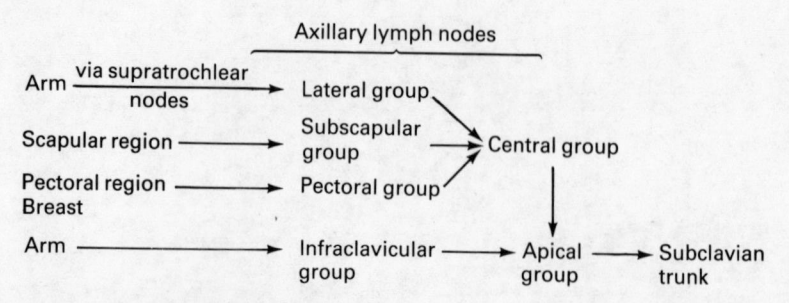

Arm — via supratrochlear nodes → Lateral group
Scapular region → Subscapular group
Pectoral region / Breast → Pectoral group
→ Central group
Arm → Infraclavicular group → Apical group → Subclavian trunk

Fig. 10 Lymphatic drainage of the upper limb.

Lymphatic system, spleen and thymus 35

Head and neck

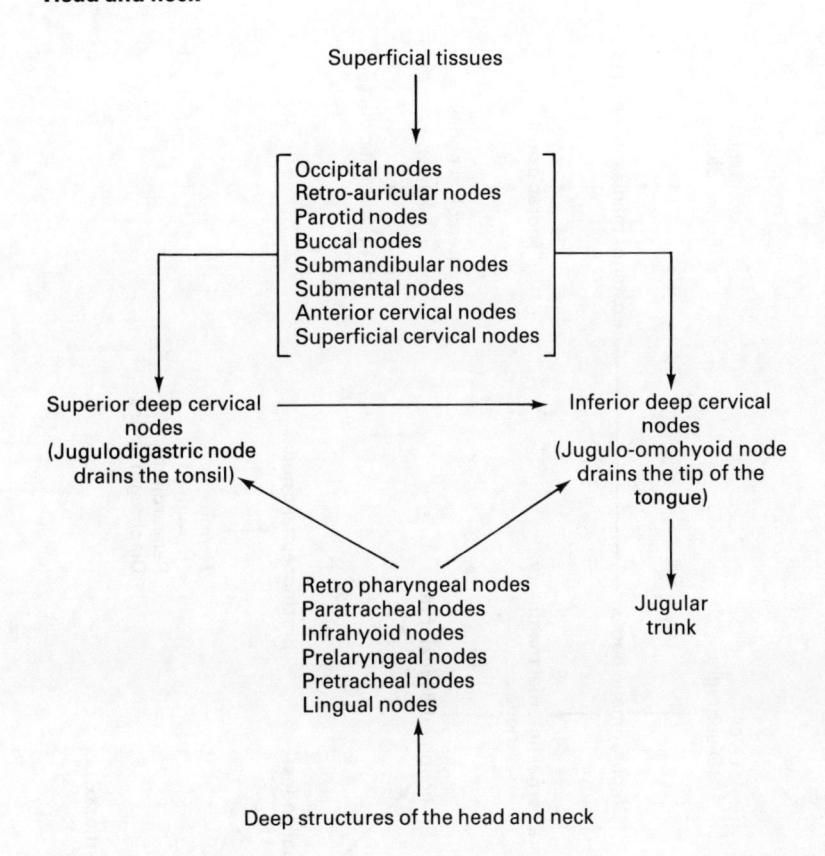

```
                    Superficial tissues
                           │
                           ▼
        ┌─────────────────────────────────────┐
        │  Occipital nodes                    │
        │  Retro-auricular nodes              │
        │  Parotid nodes                      │
        │  Buccal nodes                       │
        │  Submandibular nodes                │
        │  Submental nodes                    │
        │  Anterior cervical nodes            │
        │  Superficial cervical nodes         │
        └─────────────────────────────────────┘

Superior deep cervical    ───────▶    Inferior deep cervical
      nodes                                 nodes
(Jugulodigastric node                 (Jugulo-omohyoid node
 drains the tonsil)                    drains the tip of the
                                             tongue)
                                               │
                                               ▼
              Retro pharyngeal nodes        Jugular
              Paratracheal nodes            trunk
              Infrahyoid nodes
              Prelaryngeal nodes
              Pretracheal nodes
              Lingual nodes
                     ▲
                     │
            Deep structures of the head and neck
```

Fig. 11 Lymphatic drainage of the head and neck.

Thorax

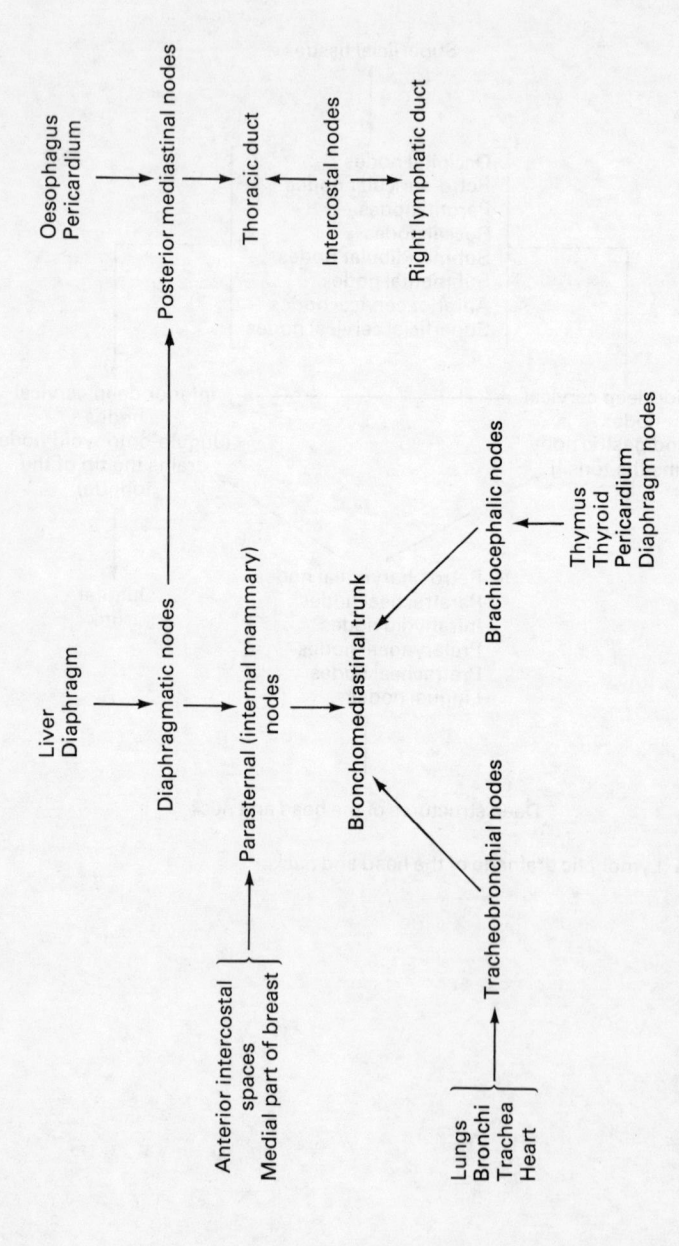

Fig. 12 Lymphatic drainage of the thorax.

Lymphatic system, spleen and thymus

SPLEEN

The spleen is an organ of the reticulo-endothelial system and is involved in phagocytosis, erythrocyte storage and immune response. It is an important haemopoetic organ in the fetus.

POSITION

The spleen lies between the 9th and 11th ribs in the left hypochondrium. Its long axis lies along the axis of the 10th rib and its inferior border extends anteriorly to the mid-axillary line.

STRUCTURE

Macroscopic
1. Anterior notch
2. Diaphragmatic surface
3. Visceral impressions
   a. gastric
   b. colic
   c. renal
4. Hilum: related to the tail of pancreas
5. Attachments
   a. gastrocolic ligaments
   b. lienorenal ligament

Microscopic
1. Outer serosal (peritoneal) layer
2. Inner fibromuscular layer: trabeculae penetrate the substance
3. Red pulp: mainly venous sinusoids
4. White pulp
   a. lymphocytes
   b. lymphoid follicles (Malpighian bodies)

BLOOD SUPPLY

Splenic artery: divides into four or five branches at hilum

VENOUS DRAINAGE

Splenic vein

LYMPH DRAINAGE

Hilum of spleen to retropancreatic nodes then to coeliac nodes

NERVE SUPPLY

Non-myelinated fibres from coeliac plexus

THYMUS

The thymus is a small gland which is the central organ of the lymphoid system.

POSITION

The thymus lies in the anterior and superior mediastinum, just behind the manubrium.

STRUCTURE

Macroscopic
1. Fibrous capsule
2. Cortex
3. Medulla

Microscopic
1. Reticular cells
2. Lymphocytes

BLOOD SUPPLY

1. Internal thoracic artery
2. Inferior thyroid artery

VENOUS DRAINAGE

1. Left brachiocephalic vein
2. Internal thoracic vein
3. Inferior thyroid vein

LYMPH DRAINAGE

1. Brachiocephalic nodes
2. Tracheobronchial nodes
3. Parasternal nodes

NERVE SUPPLY

1. Sympathetic fibres
2. Parasympathetic fibres: from vagus nerve

Nervous system

Detailed descriptions of the structures and pathways involving the brain and spinal cord are beyond the scope of this book and are only covered briefly in this chapter.

CRANIAL NERVES

There are 12 cranial nerves which are continuous with the brain and leave the skull through foramina in the base of the cranium. The motor nuclei arise from within the brain, and are connected to the motor cortex (usually contralateral) by corticonuclear fibres. The sensory part of the nerves arise from nerve cells outside the brain, grouped together as ganglia, or situated on peripheral sensory organs (e.g. nose, eye and ear). Central fibres run into the brain to sensory nuclei, and fibres proceed from here to the cortex, usually crossing to the opposite side.

The nuclei of the cranial nerves are divided into several groups. In a cross-section of the brainstem the motor (efferent) nuclei lie medial and the sensory (afferent) nuclei lie more lateral.

MOTOR (EFFERENT) NUCLEI

1. Somatic efferent: striated muscle
2. Special visceral efferent: striated muscle of pharyngeal arches
3. General visceral efferent: autonomic parasympathetic (secretomotor, motor to smooth muscle)

SENSORY (AFFERENT) NUCLEI

1. Somatic afferent: ordinary sensation
2. Special somatic afferent: hearing, sight and balance
3. Special visceral afferent: taste
4. General visceral afferent: autonomic parasympathetic (sensation)

OLFACTORY NERVE I

This nerve system is known as the rhinencephalon (see Fig. 13).

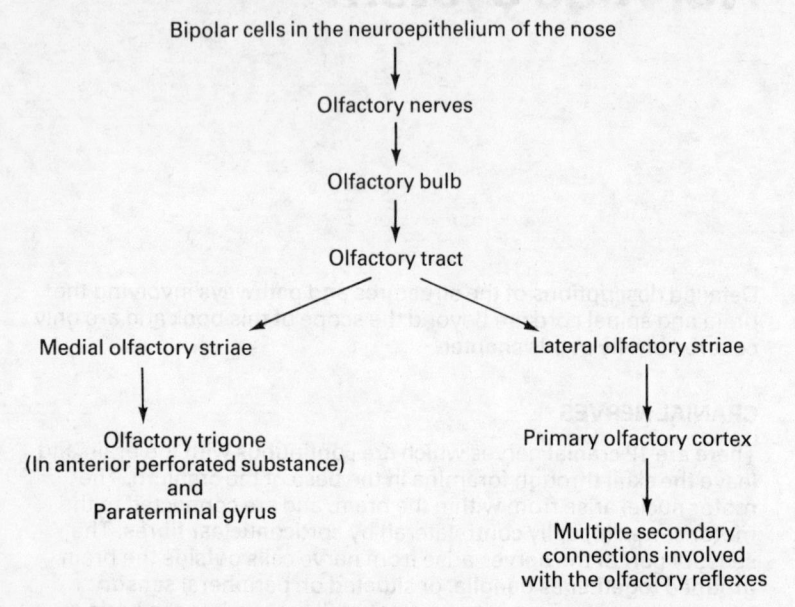

```
Bipolar cells in the neuroepithelium of the nose
                    ↓
              Olfactory nerves
                    ↓
               Olfactory bulb
                    ↓
               Olfactory tract
              ↙             ↘
  Medial olfactory striae   Lateral olfactory striae
         ↓                         ↓
   Olfactory trigone        Primary olfactory cortex
(In anterior perforated substance)   ↓
         and               Multiple secondary
   Paraterminal gyrus     connections involved
                         with the olfactory reflexes
```

Fig. 13 The olfactory nervous system.

OPTIC NERVE II

Sensory nucleus: special somatic (sight). See Figure 14.

OCCULOMOTOR NERVE III

There are two motor nuclei in the midbrain:
1. General viseral efferent (Edingher-Westphal nucleus)
2. Somatic efferent

Branches
1. Superior division
   Muscular
   (i) superior rectus
   (ii) levator palpebrae superioris
   (also supplied by sympathetic fibres)
2. Inferior division
   a. muscular
   (i) medial rectus

Nervous system 41

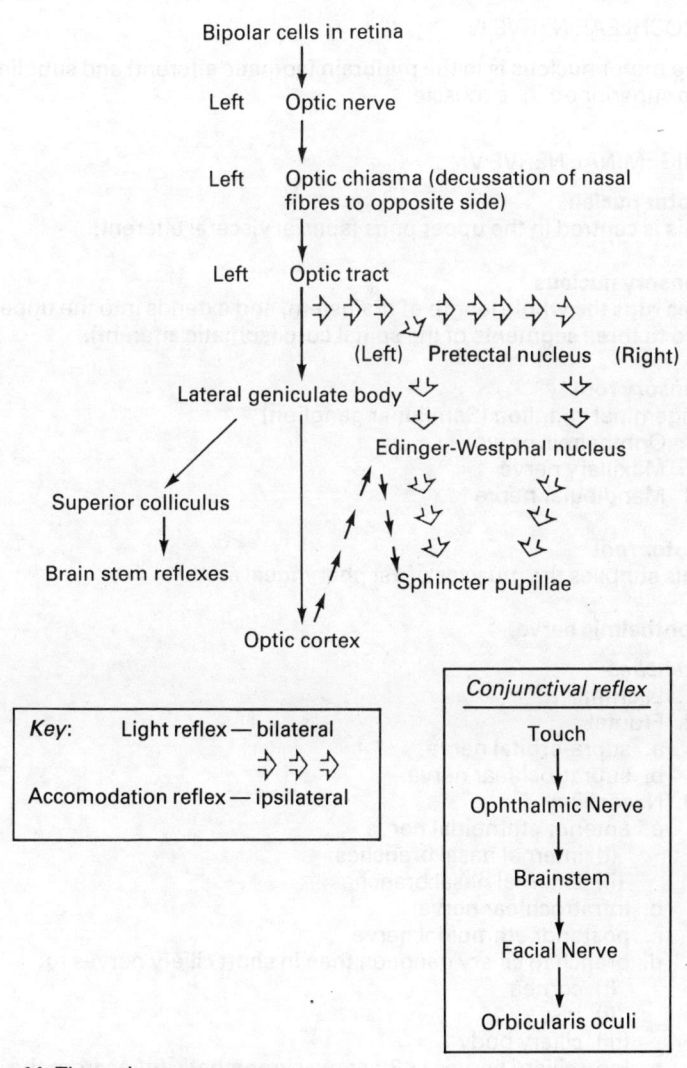

```
                    Bipolar cells in retina
                              │
            Left       Optic nerve
                              │
                              ▼
            Left       Optic chiasma (decussation of nasal
                       fibres to opposite side)
                              │
                              ▼
            Left       Optic tract
                        ⇨ ⇨ ⇨ ↙  ⇨ ⇨ ⇨ ⇨
                           (Left)  Pretectal nucleus  (Right)
          Lateral geniculate body  ⇊        ⇊
                              │    ⇊        ⇊
                              │    Edinger-Westphal nucleus
                              │    ↗↙ ⇊   ⇊
        Superior colliculus   │    ↗↙ ⇊   ⇊
                │             │       ⇊   ⇊
                ▼             │       Sphincter pupillae
        Brain stem reflexes   │
                              ▼
                        Optic cortex
```

Key:	Light reflex — bilateral ⇨ ⇨ ⇨
	Accomodation reflex — ipsilateral

```
Conjunctival reflex
─────────────────
       Touch
         │
         ▼
  Ophthalmic Nerve
         │
         ▼
     Brainstem
         │
         ▼
   Facial Nerve
         │
         ▼
  Orbicularis oculi
```

Fig. 14 The optic nervous system.

    (ii) inferior rectus
    (iii) inferior oblique
  b. parasympathetic
    to ciliary ganglion, leading to short ciliary nerves, which lead to
    — sphincter pupillae (pupil constriction)
    — ciliary muscle (accommodation)

TROCHLEAR NERVE IV

The motor nucleus is in the midbrain (somatic efferent) and supplies the superior oblique muscle.

TRIGEMINAL NERVE V

Motor nucleus
This is centred in the upper pons (special visceral efferent).

Sensory nucleus
This runs the whole length of brainstem, and extends into the upper two to three segments of the spinal cord (somatic afferent).

Sensory root
Trigeminal ganglion (Semilunar ganglion)
1. Ophthalmic nerve
2. Maxillary nerve
3. Mandibular nerve

Motor root
This supplies the muscles of 1st pharyngeal arch.

Ophthalmic nerve

Branches
1. Lacrimal
2. Frontal
   a. supra-orbital nerve
   b. supratrochlear nerve
3. Nasociliary
   a. anterior ethmoidal nerve
      (i) internal nasal branches
      (ii) external nasal branches
   b. infratrochlear nerve
   c. posterior ethmoidal nerve
   d. branch to ciliary ganglion then in short ciliary nerves to:
      (i) cornea
      (ii) iris
      (iii) ciliary body
   e. long ciliary nerves (×2): some sympathetic fibres from the cavernous plexus run in the nasociliary nerve to dilator pupillae
   Note: the short ciliary nerves contain three types of nerve fibres:
   1. Sympathetic
      a. to dilator pupillae
      b. vasomoter fibres to eyeball
   2. Sensory: to eyeball
   3. Parasympathetic: to sphincter pupillae and ciliary muscle

Maxillary nerve

Branches
1. Meningeal branch
2. Ganglionic branches
   a. pterygopalatine ganglion (sphenopalatine)
      (i) orbital branches
      (ii) palatine branches
         — greater anterior palatine nerve
         — lesser (middle and posterior) palatine nerves
      (iii) nasal branches
         — lateral posterior superior nasal nerves
         — medial posterior superior nasal nerves (one of which is the nasopalatine nerve)
      (iv) pharyngeal branch
3. Zygomatic branches
   a. zygomaticotemporal nerve
   b. zygomaticofacial nerve
4. Posterior superior alveolar nerve
5. Infraorbital nerve
   a. middle superior alveolar nerve
   b. anterior superior alveolar nerve
   c. palpebral branch
   d. nasal branch
   e. superior labial branch

Mandibular nerve

The mandibular nerve is the nerve of the 1st pharyngeal arch and carries motor and sensory fibres. The motor root joins the mandibular division of the trigeminal nerve after the trigeminal ganglion, before the nerve enters the foramen ovale. It gives off two branches from the main trunk and then divides into anterior and posterior trunks.

Branches
From main trunk
1. Meningeal branch (nervus spinosus)
2. Nerve to medial pterygoid (also supplies tensor palati and tensor tympani muscles)

The main trunk then divides into:
1. Anterior trunk
   a. buccal nerve (sensory)
   b. massateric branch: masseter
   c. temporal branches (×2): temporalis
   d. lateral pterygoid branch: lateral pterygoid
2. Posterior trunk
   a. auriculotemporal nerve
   b. lingual nerve
   c. inferior alveolar nerve: gives off the nerve to mylohyoid

ABDUCENT NERVE VI

Motor nucleus lies in the floor of the 4th ventricle (somatic efferent). The fibres leave the brain stem and follow a long course, passing over the superior border of the petrous temporal bone before entering the superior orbital fissure. This makes it particularly susceptible to compression in conditions leading to raised intracranial pressure. Paralysis of the muscle which it supplies (lateral rectus) leads to diplopia. The situation of raised intracranial pressure and resultant lateral rectus palsy is described as a 'false localizing sign'.

FACIAL NERVE VII

This is the nerve of the 2nd pharyngeal arch. It is considered to contain two cranial nerves: the 'facial nerve proper' and the nervus intermedius. They will be considered separately here.

Facial nerve
1. Motor nucleus: lower pons (special visceral efferent)
2. Sensory nucleus: upper part of nucleus of tractus solitarius

The facial nerve meets the nervus intermedius at the genicular ganglion (after which they run as one nerve).

Branches
1. Nerve to stapedius
2. Posterior Auricular nerve
3. Muscular
   a. posterior belly of diagastric
   b. stylohyoid
4. Temporozygomatic ⎫
5. Cervicofacial ⎬ rejoin in parotid gland
6. Pes Anserinus (motor branches to facial muscles)
   a. temporal branch
   b. zygomatic (upper and lower branches)
   c. buccal branch
   d. marginal mandibular branch
   e. cervical branch

The small sensory supply receives fibres from part of the skin of the external auditory meatus.

Nervus intermedius
(also referred to as the sensory root of the facial nerve)
1. Motor nucleus: superior salivatory nucleus (general visceral efferent)
2. Sensory nucleus: nucleus of the tractus solitarius (special visceral afferent — taste)

The nervus intermedius joins the facial nerve (VII) at the genicular ganglion, and thereafter they run together.

Branches
See Figure 15.

VESTIBULOCOCHLEAR NERVE VIII

This nerve consists of two sets of fibres which transmit afferent impulses from the internal ear to the brain. One set of fibres forms the vestibular nerve which with its connections is able to influence movements of the eyes and head, and muscles of the trunk and limbs in order to maintain balance.

The other set of fibres form the cochlear nerve, which transmits hearing impulses to the auditory cortices of the brain.

The central connections of both nerves are shown in Figure 16.

GLOSSOPHARYNGEAL NERVE IX

1. Sensory nuclei
    a. nucleus of tractus solitarius (special visceral afferent—taste)
    b. vital centres (special viseral sensory from carotid sinus and carotid bodies)
    c. ordinary sensation: nucleus of the spinal tract of V
2. Motor nuclei
    a. nucleus ambiguus
    b. inferior salivatory nucleus

The glossopharyngeal nerve has two sensory ganglia (the superior and inferior) on its surface at the level of the jugular foramen.

Branches
1. Tympanic nerve to tympanic plexus
    a. branch which joins the greater petrosal nerve
    b. mucous membrane of tympanic cavity, auditory tube and mastoid air cells.
    c. lesser petrosal nerve (secretomotor)
2. Lesser petrosal nerve (secretomotor): leading to otic ganglion and then to parotid gland
3. Carotid branch: descends on internal carotid artery to carotid sinus and body
4. Pharyngeal branches: pharyngeal plexus: sensory supply to mucous membrane of pharynx
5. Muscular branch: stylopharyngeus
6. Tonsillar branch
7. Lingual branches: taste and general sensation from posterior third of the tongue

VAGUS NERVE X

The vagus nerve is composed of motor and sensory fibres, and has an extensive course through the neck and thorax to the abdomen.

46 Aids to anatomy

(a) Greater superficial petrosal nerve → Vidian nerve → Pterygopalatine ganglion → Secretomotor fibres run with the branches of pterygopalatine ganglion { Orbital, Palatine, Nasal, Pharyngeal }

Deep petrosal nerve (sympathetic fibres from carotid plexus)

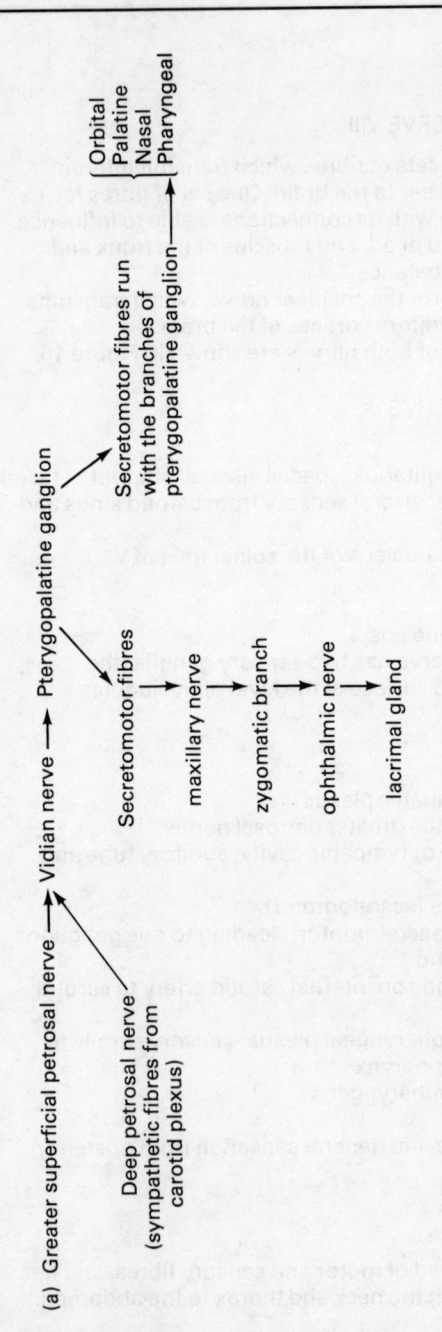

Secretomotor fibres → maxillary nerve → zygomatic branch → ophthalmic nerve → lacrimal gland

(b) Chordae Tympani → joins lingual nerve ↔ Taste fibres from anterior two-thirds of the tongue / Submandibular ganglion (secretomotor fibres) → Sublingual gland, Submandibular gland

Fig. 15 Branches of the nervus intermedius.

Nervous system 47

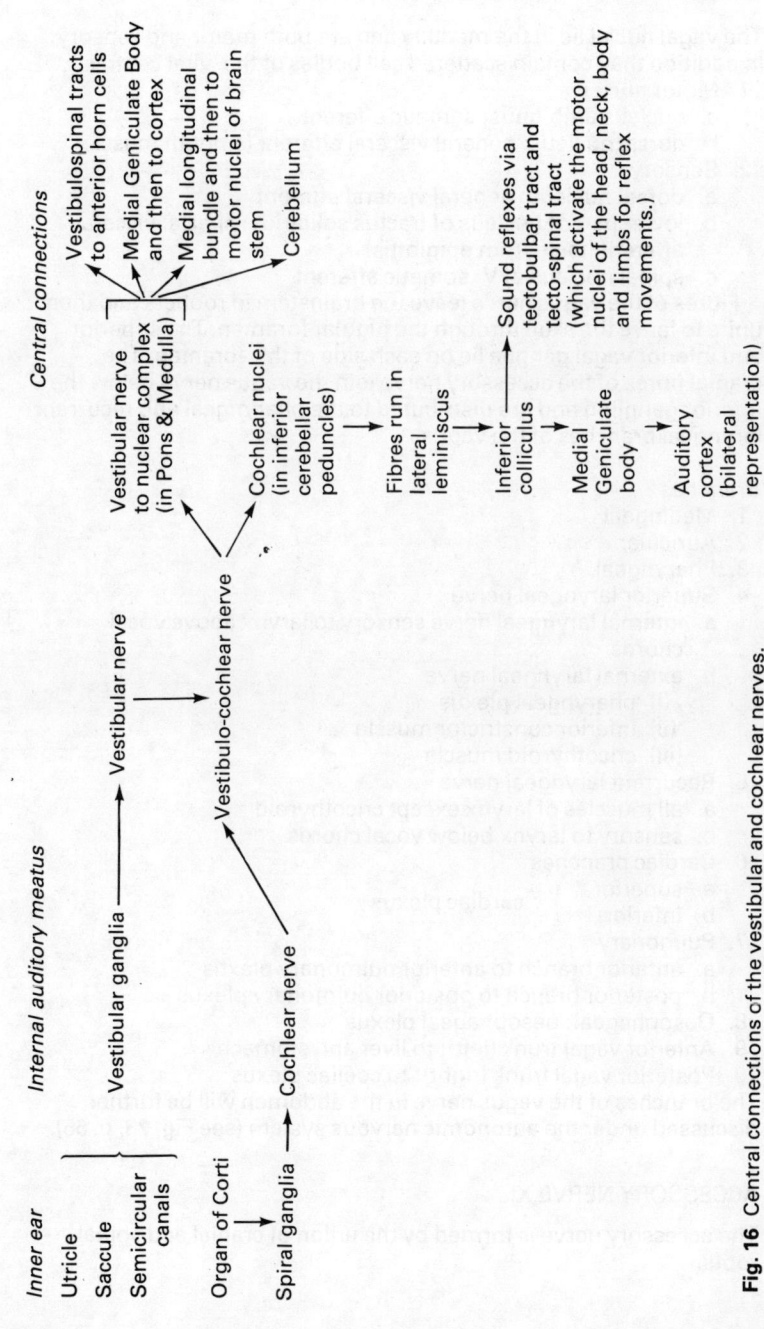

Inner ear	Internal auditory meatus		Central connections
Utricle			Vestibulospinal tracts to anterior horn cells
Saccule	Vestibular ganglia → Vestibular nerve →	Vestibular nerve to nuclear complex (in Pons & Medulla)	Medial Geniculate Body and then to cortex
Semicircular canals			Medial longitudinal bundle and then to motor nuclei of brain stem
			Cerebellum
Organ of Corti → Spiral ganglia → Cochlear nerve →	Vestibulo-cochlear nerve	Cochlear nuclei (in inferior cerebellar peduncles) → Fibres run in lateral lemniscus → Inferior colliculus → Medial Geniculate body → Auditory cortex (bilateral representation)	Sound reflexes via tectobulbar tract and tecto-spinal tract (which activate the motor nuclei of the head, neck, body and limbs for reflex movements.)

Fig. 16 Central connections of the vestibular and cochlear nerves.

The vagal nuclei lie in the medulla and are both motor and sensory. In addition they contain scattered cell bodies of the 'vital centres'.
1. Motor nuclei
   a. nucleus ambiguus: somatic efferent
   b. dorsal nucleus: general visceral efferent (smooth muscle)
2. Sensory
   a. dorsal nucleus: general visceral afferent
   b. lower part of nucleus of tractus solitarius: special visceral afferent (taste from epiglottis)
   c. spinal nucleus of V: somatic afferent

Fibres of the vagus nerve leave the brainstem in rootlets and then unite to leave the skull through the jugular foramen. The superior and inferior vagal ganglia lie on each side of this foramen. The cranial fibres of the accessory nerve join the vagus nerve below the inferior ganglion and are distributed to the pharyngeal and recurrent laryngeal branches of the vagus.

Branches
1. Meningeal
2. Auricular
3. Pharyngeal
4. Superior laryngeal nerve
   a. internal laryngeal nerve sensory to larynx above vocal chords
   b. external laryngeal nerve
      (i) pharyngeal plexus
      (ii) inferior constrictor muscle
      (iii) cricothyroid muscle
5. Recurrent laryngeal nerve
   a. all muscles of larynx except cricothyroid
   b. sensory to larynx below vocal chords
6. Cardiac branches
   a. superior } cardiac plexus
   b. inferior }
7. Pulmonary
   a. anterior branch to anterior pulmonary plexus
   b. posterior branch to posterior pulmonary plexus
8. Oesophageal: oesophageal plexus
9. Anterior vagal trunk (left): to liver and stomach
10. Posterior vagal trunk (right): to coeliac plexus

The branches of the vagus nerve in the abdomen will be further discussed under the autonomic nervous system (see Fig. 23, p. 65).

ACCESSORY NERVE XI

The accessory nerve is formed by the union of cranial and spinal roots.

Cranial root
Motor nuclei: nucleus ambiguus in the medulla.

Branches
Distributed in the pharyngeal and recurrent laryngeal branches of the Vagus nerve.

Spinal root
Spinal nucleus in anterior grey columns of the upper spinal cord (C1–5).
The fibres leave the spinal cord between the ventral and dorsal nerve roots. They unite and ascend through the foramen magnum, behind the vertebral artery. The spinal root joins the cranial root in the jugular foramen. The fibres in the cranial root join the vagus nerve below the inferior vagal ganglion.

Branches
1. Sternocleidomastoid muscle
2. Trapezius muscle

HYPOGLOSSAL NERVE XII

This is the motor nerve to the tongue.

Motor nucleus — Hypoglossal nucleus in medulla.
The fibres emerge from the surface of the medulla in a series of rootlets between the pyramid and olive. They join into two roots that enter the hypoglossal (anterior condylar) canal in the occipital bone, becoming one nerve in this canal.
   The hypoglossal nerve communicates with the vagus, and the 1st and 2nd cervical and lingual nerves.

Branches
1. Meningeal branch
2. Descending branch: this is the upper root of the ansa cervicalis and only contains fibres from the first cervical nerve (C1)
3. Nerve to thyrohyoid (C1 fibres)
4. Muscular branches to the tongue:
    a. styloglossus
    b. hyoglossus
    c. geniohyoid (C1 fibres)
    d. genioglossus
    e. intrinsic muscles of the tongue

SPINAL NERVES

The spinal nerves are somatic and consist of anterior and posterior primary rami. They sequentially supply the muscles and skin of the body wall and limbs, extending from C1 to the coccygeal nerves. Although essentially somatic, these nerves also carry autonomic fibres; these are discussed under the autonomic nervous system (see p. 60). For a typical spinal nerve, see Figure 17.

POSTERIOR PRIMARY RAMI OF SPINAL NERVES

The posterior primary rami divide into medial and lateral branches which supply the erector spinae group of muscles and the overlying skin.

The posterior primary rami of the upper three cervical nerves are:
1. C1 — suboccipital nerve: muscular to suboccipital muscles
2. C2 — greater occipital nerve: sensory to scalp
3. C3 — 3rd occipital nerve: sensory to occipital region

The nerves from C2 and C3 are actually from the medial branch of the posterior primary rami.

ANTERIOR PRIMARY RAMI OF SPINAL NERVES

The anterior primary rami sequentially supply the skin and muscles of the rest of the body wall and limbs. They run in the neurovascular plane between the inner and innermost layer of muscles. In the region of the upper and lower limbs they form plexuses, from which are derived the nerves to that limb.

The plexuses formed by the anterior primary rami of spinal nerves are:
1. C1–4: cervical plexus
2. C5–T1: brachial plexus
3. L1–L4: lumbar plexus
4. L4–S3: lumbosacral plexus

Cervical plexus

Nerves from roots
1. C1
   a. communicates with vagus nerve
   b. superior root of ansa cervicalis
   c. muscular to:
      (i) rectus capitis anterior
      (ii) longus capitis
      (iii) rectus lateralis

Nervous system 51

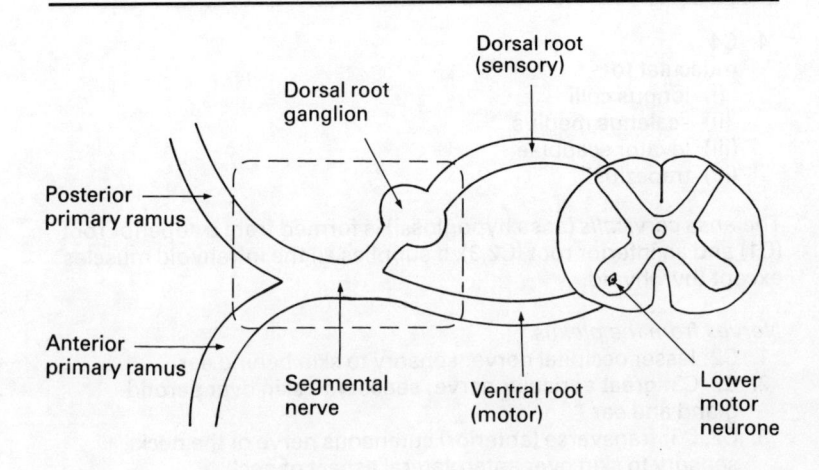

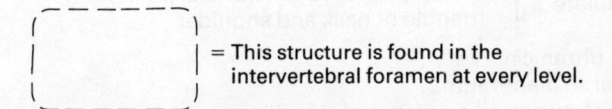

Fig. 17 A typical spinal nerve.

(dashed box) = This structure is found in the intervertebral foramen at every level.

2. C2
    a. inferior root of ansa cervicalis
    b. muscular to:
        (i) longus capitis
        (ii) longus colli
        (iii) sternocleidomastoid*
3. C3
    a. inferior root of ansa cervicalis
    b. muscular to:
        (i) longus capitis
        (ii) longus colli
        (iii) scalenus medius
        (iv) levator scapulae
        (v) trapezius*

* The branches to trapezius and sternocleidomastoid are probably only proprioceptive

4. C4
    muscular to:
      (i) longus colli
      (ii) scalenus medius
      (iii) levator scapulae
      (iv) trapezius*

The *ansa cervicalis* (ansa hypoglossi) is formed from a superior root (C1) and an inferior root (C2,3). It supplies all the infrahyoid muscles except thyrohyoid.

Nerves from the plexus
1. C2: lesser occipital nerve: sensory to skin behind ear
2. C2, C3: great auricular nerve: sensory to skin over parotid gland and ear
3. C2, C3: transverse (anterior) cutaneous nerve of the neck: sensory to skin over anterolateral aspect of neck
4. C3, C4: supraclavicular nerves
    a. medial
    b. intermediate } sensory to skin over clavicle, posterior triangle of neck and shoulder
    c. lateral
5. C3, C4, C5: phrenic nerve
    a. muscular to diaphragm
    b. sensory to surrounding pleura and peritoneum

The C5 of the phrenic nerve may arise separately as the accessory phrenic nerve from a branch of the nerve to subclavius.

Brachial plexus

Branches from roots
1. C5
    a. dorsal scapular nerve: muscular to rhomboid muscles
    b. muscular to scaleni
    c. branch to phrenic nerve
2. C6, C7, C8: muscular to scaleni
3. T1: first intercostal nerve
4. C5, C6, C7: long thoracic nerve (of Bell): muscular to serratus anterior

Branches from trunks
1. C5, C6: nerve to subclavius
2. C5, C6: suprascapular nerve: muscular to supraspinatus and infraspinatus

---

* The branches to trapezius and sternocleidomastoid are probably only proprioceptive

Branches from cords

Lateral cord
1. C5, C6, C7: lateral pectoral nerve: pectoral muscles
2. C5, C6, C7: musculocutaneous nerve
   a. biceps, brachialis,
   b. coracobrachialis
   c. lateral cutaneous nerve of forearm
3. C6, C7: lateral root of median nerve

Medial cord
1. C8, T1: medial root of median nerve

   Branches of median nerve
   Muscular to:
   a. pronator teres
   b. flexor carpi radialis
   c. palmaris longus
   d. flexor digitorum superficialis
   e. flexor pollicis brevis
   f. abductor pollicis brevis
   g. opponens pollicis
   Articular to: elbow
   Anterior interosseous nerve
   a. flexor pollicis longus
   b. flexor digitorum profundus
   c. pronator quadratus
   d. articular to wrist and carpus
   Cutaneous: skin over palm
   Digital nerves
   a. skin over thenar eminence
   b. skin over radial three and a half digits
   c. muscular to 1st and 2nd lumbricals

2. C8, T1: medial pectoral nerve: pectoral muscles
3. C8, T1: medial cutaneous nerve of forearm and arm
4. C7, C8, T1: ulnar nerve
   a. articular—elbow
   b. muscular
      (i) flexor carpi ulnaris
      (ii) flexor digitorum profundus
      (iii) palmaris brevis
      (iv) abductor digiti minimi
      (v) flexor digiti minimi
      (vi) opponens digiti minimi
      (vii) 3rd and 4th lumbricals and all interossei
      (viii) adductor pollicis
   c. cutaneous: skin of palm
   d. digital nerves; skin over ulnar one and a half digits and ulnar side of dorsum of hand

Posterior cord
1. C5, C6: upper subscapular nerve: subscapularis
2. C6, C7, C8: thoracodorsal nerve: latissimus dorsi
3. C5, C6: lower subscapular nerve: muscular to
    (i) subscapularis
    (ii) teres major
4. C5, C6: axillary nerve
    a. Anterior branch
        (i) deltoid muscle
        (ii) sensory to skin over deltoid
    b. Posterior branch
        (i) teres minor
        (ii) deltoid
        (iii) upper lateral cutaneous nerve of the arm
5. C5, C6, C7, C8, T1: radial nerve

Branches:
1. Muscular
    a. triceps
    b. anconeus
    c. brachioradialis
    d. extensor carpi radialis longus
    e. brachialis
2. Posterior cutaneous nerve of arm
3. Lower lateral cutaneous nerve of arm
4. Posterior cutaneous nerve of forearm
5. Dorsal digital nerves: sensory to skin over dorsum of hand and fingers
6. Articular branches to elbow joint
7. Posterior interosseous nerve
    a. extensor carpi radialis brevis
    b. supinator
    c. extensor digitorum
    d. extensor digiti minimi
    e. extensor carpi ulnaris
    f. extensor pollicis longus
    g. extensor indicis
    h. abductor pollicis longus
    i. articular branches to carpus
    j. extensor pollicis brevis

Thoracic (intercostal) nerves
They run along the superior aspect of the intercostal space between the inner and innermost intercostal muscles, just below each rib.

Branches
1. Collateral branch: runs along the inferior aspect of the intercostal space
2. Lateral cutaneous branch

3. Anterior cutaneous branch
   4. Muscular branches to:
      a. intercostal muscles
      b. muscles of anterior abdominal wall

Additional information
   1. T1: The anterior primary ramus divides
      1. Branch to brachial plexus
      2. 1st intercostal nerve
   2. T2: lateral cutaneous branch is called the intercostobrachial nerve and supplies skin over upper half of medial aspect of arm
   3. T3: lateral cutaneous branch forms the 2nd intercostobrachial nerve and supplies skin of axilla
   4. T2–6: anterior cutaneous branches form the anterior cutaneous nerves of the thorax
   5. T7–11: these intercostal nerves continue below the costal margin supplying the skin and muscles of the anterior abdominal wall
   6. T10: supplies the skin over the umbilicus
   7. T12: subcostal nerve

Lumbar plexus
The lumbar plexus, formed from the ventral rami of the first four lumbar nerves, divides into dorsal and ventral divisions after giving off several branches from the nerve roots.

Branches from roots
   1. T12–L4: to quadratus lumborum
   2. L1: to psoas minor
   3. L2, L3, L4: to psoas major
   4. L2, L3: to iliacus
   5. L1: iliohypogastric nerve
      a. skin over abdomen above pubis
      b. skin over side of buttock (anteriorly)
   6. L1: ilioinguinal nerve
      a. skin over superomedial part of thigh
      b. skin over root of penis
      c. skin over scrotum
      d. skin over
         (i) mons pubis
         (ii) labia majora
   7. L1, L2: genitofemoral nerve
      a. genital branch
         (i) cremaster muscle
         (ii) skin of scrotum
         (iii) skin over mons pubis
         (iv) skin over labia majora
      b. femoral branch: skin over upper part of femoral triangle

Dorsal division of lumbar plexus
1. L2, L3: lateral cutaneous nerve of thigh
   a. anterior branch
   b. posterior branch
2. L2, L3, L4: femoral nerve
   a. in abdomen
      (i) pectineus
      (ii) iliacus
   b. in thigh
      (i) anterior division
         — intermediate cutaneous nerve of thigh
         — medial cutaneous nerve of thigh
         — sartorius
      (ii) posterior division
         — saphenous nerve
         — quadriceps femoris
         — knee joint

Ventral divisions of lumbar plexus
1. L2–4: obturator nerve
   a. anterior branch
      (i) cutaneous branch
      (ii) adductor longus
      (iii) gracilis
      (iv) adductor brevis
      (v) pectineus
   b. posterior branch
      (i) obturator externus
      (ii) adductor magnus
      (iii) adductor brevis
      (iv) articular to knee
2. L3, L4: accessory obturator nerve
   a. pectineus
   b. hip joint
3. L4, L5: lumbosacral nerve: continues into sacral plexus

Subsartorial plexus
This is a plexus of cutaneous nerves beneath the sartorius muscle formed from   1. Branches of the saphenous nerve
   2. Medial cutaneous nerve of thigh
   3. Anterior branch of obturator nerve
It gives off branches which supply the medial side of the thigh.

Patellar plexus
This is a cutaneous nerve plexus formed by branches from:
1. Saphenous nerve
2. Anterior branch of lateral cutaneous nerve of thigh
3. Anterior division of femoral nerve
It supplies the skin over the patella.

Sacral plexus
1. L4, L5 from lumbosacral trunk
2. S1, S2, S3

Ventral divisions
1. L4, L5, S1 muscular to
   a. quadratus femoris
   b. gemellus inferior
2. L5, S1, S2 muscular to
   a. obturator internus
   b. gemellus superior
3. L4, L5, S1, S2, S3: tibial branch of sciatic nerve
4. S2, S3, S4: pudendal nerve
5. S4: muscular to
   a. levator ani
   b. coccygeus
   c. external anal sphincter
6. S2, S3, S4: pelvic splanchnic nerves: supply pelvic viscera
7. S2, S3: posterior femoral cutaneous nerve
   a. perineum
   b. back of thigh
   c. calf

Dorsal divisions
1. S1, S2: posterior femoral cutaneous nerve: sensory to
   a. buttock
   b. perineum
   c. back of thigh
   d. calf
2. S1, S2: muscular to piriformis
3. L4, L5, S1: superior gluteal nerve: gluteus medius and minimus
4. L5, S1, S2: inferior gluteal nerve: gluteus maximus
5. L4, L5: common peroneal branch of sciatic nerve
6. S2, S3: perforating cutaneous nerve: skin over gluteus maximus

Pudendal nerve (S2, S3, S4)
1. Inferior rectal nerve
   a. external anal sphincter
   b. lower part of anal mucosa
   c. perianal skin
2. Perineal nerve
   a. sensory to:
      (i) lower part of vagina
      (ii) skin of scrotum/labia majora
      (iii) urethra
   b. muscular to:
      (i) transversus perinei superficialis
      (ii) bulbospongiosus
      (iii) ischiocavernosus

(iv) transversus perinei profundus
(v) sphincter urethrae
(vi) external anal sphincter
(vii) levator ani
3. Dorsal nerve of penis to
(i) corpus cavernosum
(ii) glans penis
Dorsal nerve of clitoris: sensory to clitoris

Sciatic nerve (L4, L5, S1, S2, S3)
1. Articular: hip joint
2. Muscular
   a. biceps femoris
   b. semitendinosus
   c. semimembranosus
   d. adductor magnus (ischial head)

Tibial nerve (L4, L5, S1, S2, S3)
1. Articular: knee and ankle
2. Muscular
   a. gastrocnemius
   b. plantaris
   c. soleus
   d. popliteus
   e. tibialis posterior
   f. flexor digitorum longus
   g. flexor hallucis longus
3. Sural Nerve: skin over lateral part of leg and foot up to little toe
4. Medial calcanean branches: skin of heel and medial part of sole
5. Medial plantar nerve
   a. cutaneous to sole of foot
   b. abductor hallucis
   c. flexor digitorum brevis
   d. first lumbrical
   e. articular to tarsus and metatarsus
   f. three plantar digital nerves
      (i) cutaneous to medial three and a half toes
      (ii) flexor hallucis brevis
6. Lateral plantar nerve
   a. flexor digitorum accessorius
   b. abductor digiti minimi
   c. flexor digiti minimi brevis
   d. interossei
   e. adductor hallucis
   f. 2nd–4th lumbricals
   g. skin over lateral one and a half digits

Common peroneal nerve (L4, L5, S1, S2 Lateral popliteal nerve)
1. Articular: knee joint
2. Cutaneous
   a. lateral cutaneous nerve of calf
   b. sural communicating branch
3. Deep peroneal nerve
   a. tibialis anterior
   b. extensor digitorum longus
   c. peroneus tertius
   d. extensor hallucis longus
   e. articular to ankle joint
   f. lateral terminal branch
      (i) extensor digitorum brevis
      (ii) interosseus branches to tarsus and metatarsophalangeal joints
   g. medial terminal branch
      (i) two dorsal digital nerves
      (ii) interosseus branch to 1st metatarsophalangeal joint
4. Superficial peroneal nerve (musculocutaneous nerve)
   a. muscular to peroneus longus and peroneus brevis
   b. cutaneous to skin over lower leg
   c. dorsal digital nerves: skin over dorsal surfaces of all toes except:

Table 1 Segmental innervation of joint movements

Joint	Movement	Nerve
Shoulder	Abduction and lateral rotation	C5
	Adduction and medial rotation	C6, C7, C8
Elbow	Flexion	C(5) 6
	Extension	C7(8)
Forearm	Supination	C6
	Pronation	C7, C8
Wrist	Flexion and Extension	C6, C7
Hand	Long flexors and extensors	C7, C8
	Intrinsic muscles	C8, T1
Hip	Flexion, adduction, medial rotation	L1, L2, L3
	Extension, abduction, lateral rotation	L5, S1
Knee	Extension	L3, L4
	Flexion	L5, S1
Ankle	Dorsiflexion	L4, L5
	Plantar flexion	S1, S2
Foot	Inversion	L4, L5
	Eversion	L5, S1

Reflexes:

Ankle	S1, S2
Knee	L3, L4
Biceps	C5, C6
Triceps	C7, C8
Wrist	C5, C6

(i) lateral side of little toe (sural nerve)
(ii) adjoining sides of great and 2nd toe (branches from deep peroneal nerve)

AUTONOMIC NERVOUS SYSTEM

The autonomic nervous system differs from the somatic nervous system in that it is primarily 'involuntary' and because the efferent nerve fibres synapse outside the central nervous system. The sympathetic fibres usually synapse in ganglia of the sympathetic chain and the parasympathetic fibres synapse in ganglia close to the end organ. All synapses occur in 'ganglia' and there are pre- and post-ganglionic fibres for the autonomic nerves. The former are myelinated and the latter non-myelinated.

The afferent pathways of the autonomic nervous system resemble those of the somatic, with unipolar cell bodies in the cranial and spinal ganglia. The central processes accompany the somatic afferent fibres through the dorsal root ganglion to the central nervous system.

The autonomic nervous system is composed of sympathetic and parasympathetic nerves. The main actions are outlined in Table 2.

SYMPATHETIC NERVOUS SYSTEM
See Figure 18.

Sympathetic chain
The sympathetic chain is made up of many ganglia, and lies on each side of the vertebral column from the base of the skull (superior cervical ganglia) to the coccyx (ganglion impar). It lies anterior to the transverse processes of the cervical and lumbar vertebrae, anterior to the heads of the ribs in the thorax, and in the pelvis medial to the anterior sacral foramina (see Fig. 19).

Position of the main sympathetic plexuses
1. Cardiac plexus: base of heart below arch of aorta
2. Pulmonary plexus: root of the lungs
3. Coeliac plexus: coeliac axis and origin of superior mesenteric artery
4. Superior hypogastric plexus: anterior to the bifurcation of the aorta
5. Inferior hypogastric plexus: lateral sides of the rectum

Post-ganglionic sympathetic nerve fibres are distributed to the viscera either directly or along branches of the arterial supply.

Table 2 Main actions of the sympathetic and parasympathetic nerves of the autonomic nervous system

Sympathetic activity	Parasympathetic activity
Vascular	
Peripheral vasoconstriction	
Splanchnic vasoconstriction	
Salivary gland vasoconstriction	Salivary gland vasodilation
Coronary artery dilation	
Increased heart rate	Decreased heart rate
Renin release	
Visceral	
Bronchial dilatation	Bronchoconstriction
Decreased bronchial secretions	Increased bronchial secretions
Pupil dilatation	Pupil constriction
Increase skin sweating	
Decreased gut motility	Increased gut mobility
Contraction of sphincters	Relaxation of sphincters
	Contraction of bladder detrusor muscle
	Erection in male
	Contraction of gallbladder
Metabolic	
Lipolysis	Increased pancreatic exocrine secretion
Glycogenolysis	
Gluconeogenesis	
Adrenaline release from adrenal medulla	

PARASYMPATHETIC NERVOUS SYSTEM

The parasympathetic nervous system is secretomotor to glands and motor to non-striated muscle.

The parasympathetic nervous system has cranial and sacral parts.

Cranial parasympathetic outflow
(See Figs. 20–23).

Sacral parasympathetic outflow
See Figure 24.

All the parasympathetic pre-ganglionic nerve fibres synapse in ganglia near the end organs. In the head these are:
1. Ciliary ganglia
2. Pterygopalatine ganglia
3. Submandibular ganglia
4. Otic ganglia

In the rest of the body these ganglia are much smaller and are found in the surface of the end organs.

62 Aids to anatomy

Lateral horn of grey matter of spinal cord (T1–L2)
↓
Pre-ganglionic fibres (myelinated) leave spinal cord in anterior primary ramus
↓
Enter ganglion of sympathetic chain at that level through white ramus comminicantes

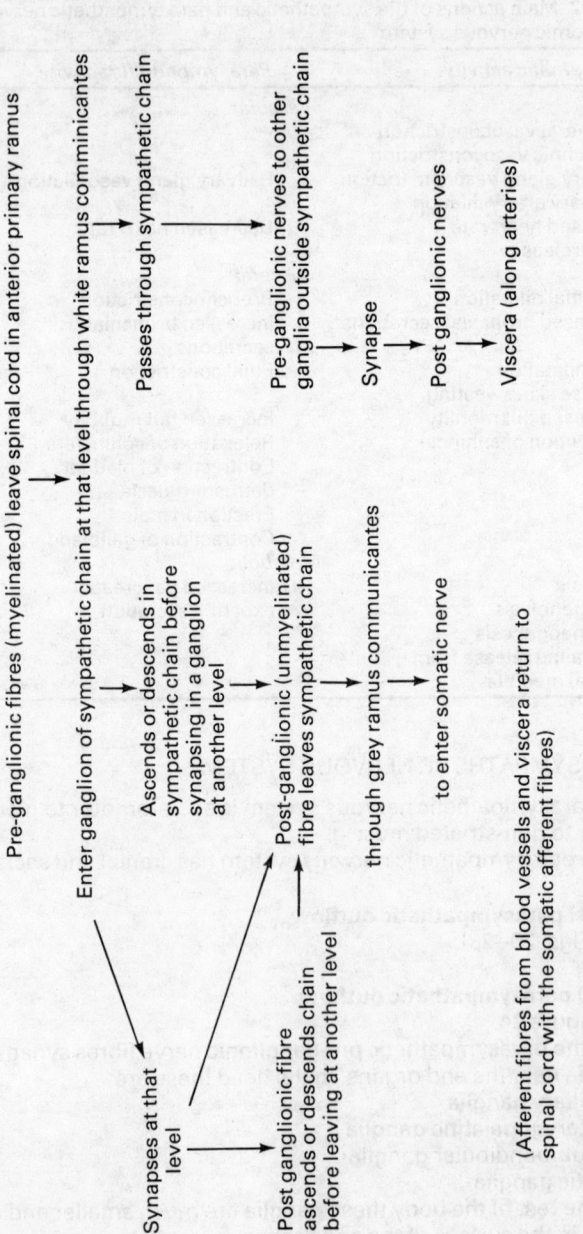

From here:
- Passes through sympathetic chain → Pre-ganglionic nerves to other ganglia outside sympathetic chain → Synapse → Post ganglionic nerves → Viscera (along arteries)
- Ascends or descends in sympathetic chain before synapsing in a ganglion at another level → Post-ganglionic (unmyelinated) fibre leaves sympathetic chain → through grey ramus communicantes → to enter somatic nerve
- Synapses at that level → Post ganglionic fibre ascends or descends chain before leaving at another level ↗ (to post-ganglionic fibre above)

(Afferent fibres from blood vessels and viscera return to spinal cord with the somatic afferent fibres)

Fig. 18 The sympathetic nervous system.

Nervous system

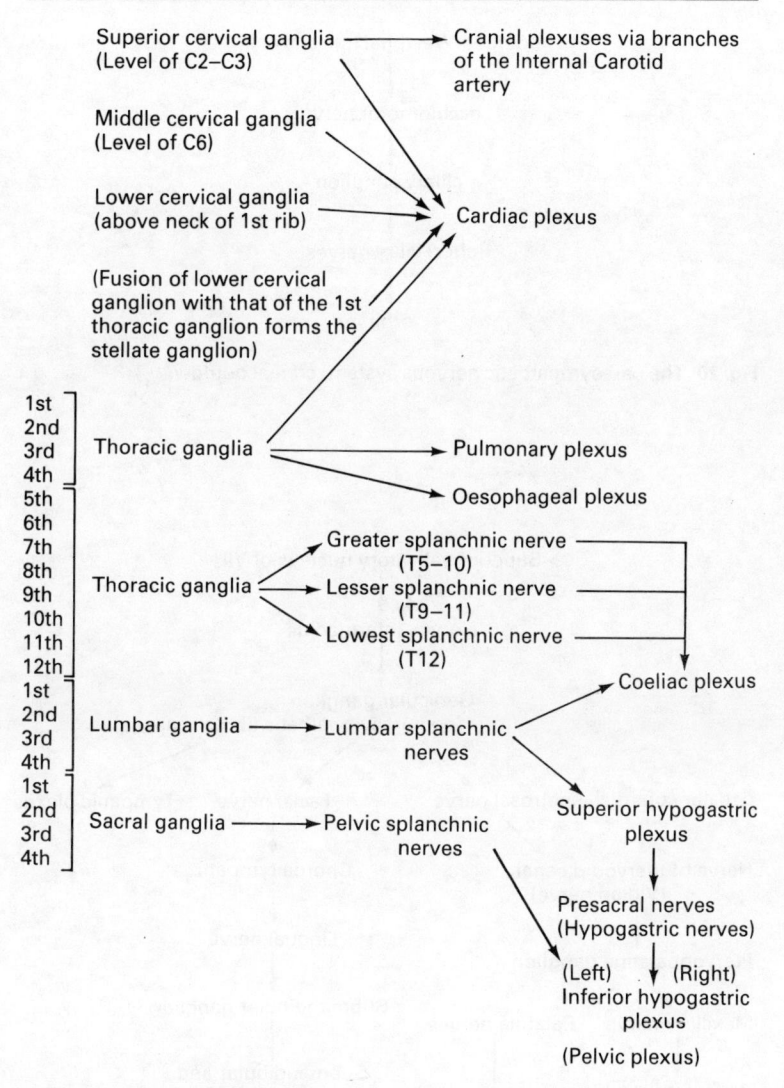

```
Superior cervical ganglia ─────▶ Cranial plexuses via branches
(Level of C2–C3)                  of the Internal Carotid
                                  artery
Middle cervical ganglia
(Level of C6)

Lower cervical ganglia
(above neck of 1st rib) ──────▶ Cardiac plexus

(Fusion of lower cervical
ganglion with that of the 1st
thoracic ganglion forms the
stellate ganglion)

1st ┐
2nd │
3rd │ Thoracic ganglia ──────▶ Pulmonary plexus
4th ┘                    ╲──▶ Oesophageal plexus
5th ┐
6th │
7th │                    ┌─▶ Greater splanchnic nerve
8th │ Thoracic ganglia ──┼─▶  (T5–10)
9th │                    ├─▶ Lesser splanchnic nerve
10th│                    │    (T9–11)
11th│                    └─▶ Lowest splanchnic nerve
12th┘                         (T12)
                                                ▶ Coeliac plexus
1st ┐
2nd │ Lumbar ganglia ──▶ Lumbar splanchnic
3rd │                     nerves
4th ┘
1st ┐                                    Superior hypogastric
2nd │                                    plexus
3rd │ Sacral ganglia ──▶ Pelvic splanchnic         │
4th ┘                     nerves                   ▼
                                         Presacral nerves
                                         (Hypogastric nerves)
                                    (Left)  ▼  (Right)
                                    Inferior hypogastric
                                    plexus
                                    (Pelvic plexus)
```

Fig. 19 The sympathetic chain.

The splanchnic nerves are pre-ganglionic fibres and synapse in ganglia of the coeliac, superior and inferior hypogastric plexuses.

64 Aids to anatomy

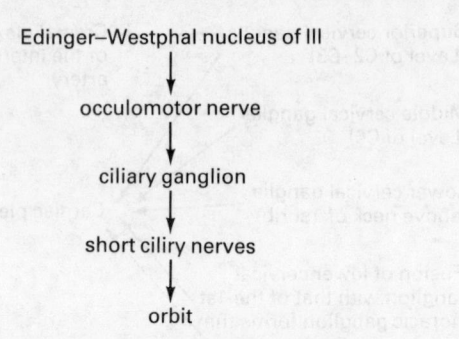

```
Edinger–Westphal nucleus of III
            ↓
      occulomotor nerve
            ↓
       ciliary ganglion
            ↓
     short ciliary nerves
            ↓
           orbit
```

Fig. 20 The parasympathetic nervous system: cranial outflow.

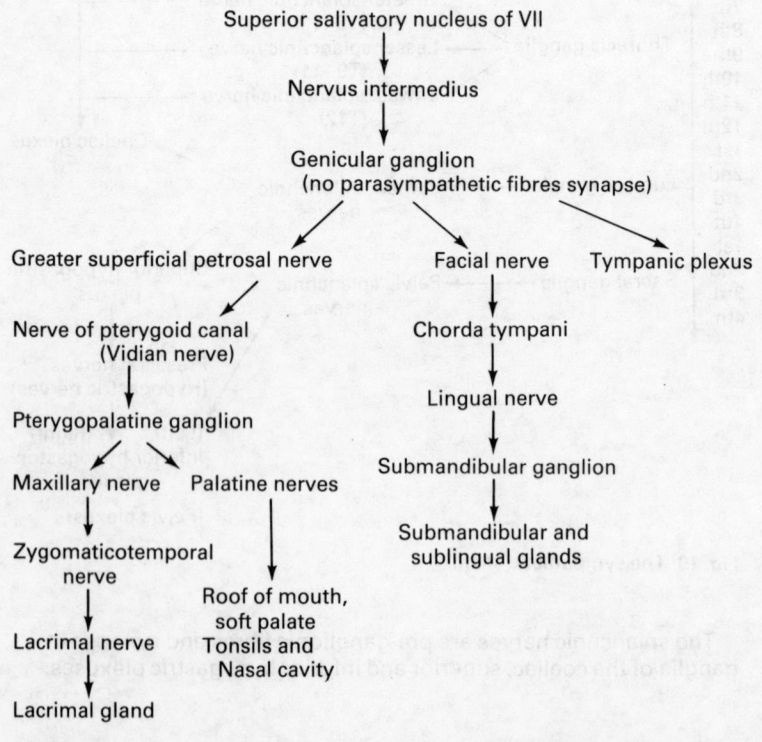

```
              Superior salivatory nucleus of VII
                          ↓
                   Nervus intermedius
                          ↓
                   Genicular ganglion
              (no parasympathetic fibres synapse)
              ↙              ↓              ↘
Greater superficial      Facial nerve      Tympanic plexus
 petrosal nerve               ↓
      ↓                  Chorda tympani
Nerve of pterygoid canal      ↓
  (Vidian nerve)         Lingual nerve
      ↓                       ↓
Pterygopalatine ganglion  Submandibular ganglion
   ↙        ↘                 ↓
Maxillary  Palatine       Submandibular and
 nerve     nerves         sublingual glands
   ↓          ↓
Zygomaticotemporal
  nerve
   ↓       Roof of mouth,
Lacrimal    soft palate
 nerve     Tonsils and
   ↓       Nasal cavity
Lacrimal gland
```

Fig. 21 The parasympathetic nervous system: cranial outflow.

Nervous system 65

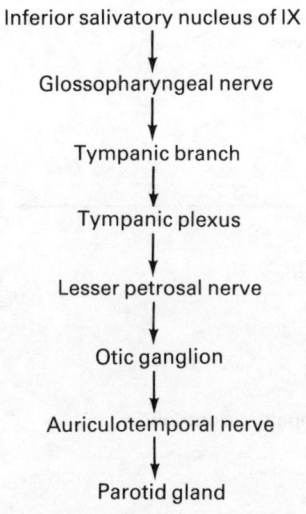

```
Inferior salivatory nucleus of IX
              ↓
   Glossopharyngeal nerve
              ↓
       Tympanic branch
              ↓
       Tympanic plexus
              ↓
     Lesser petrosal nerve
              ↓
         Otic ganglion
              ↓
    Auriculotemporal nerve
              ↓
         Parotid gland
```

Fig. 22 The parasympathetic nervous system: cranial outflow.

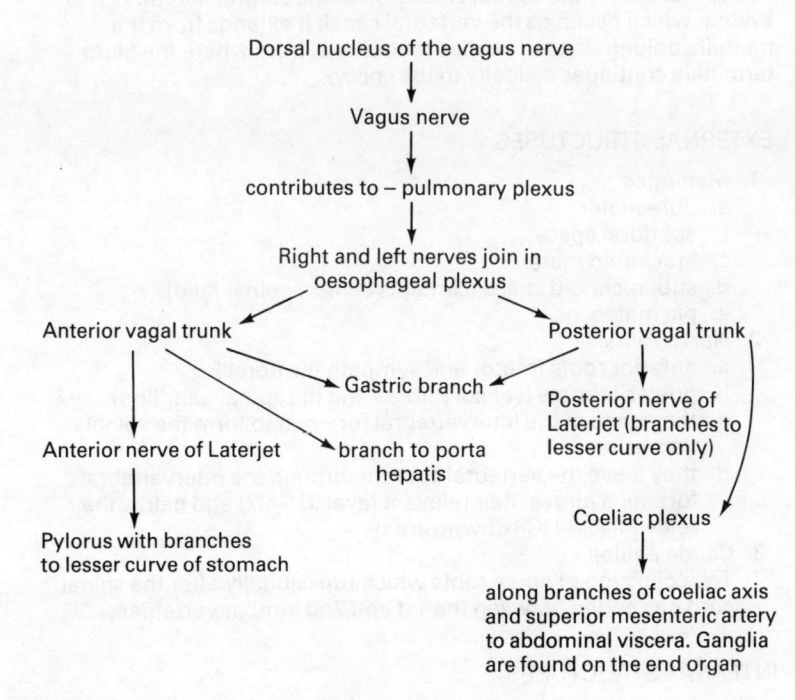

```
Dorsal nucleus of the vagus nerve
              ↓
          Vagus nerve
              ↓
   contributes to – pulmonary plexus
              ↓
   Right and left nerves join in
        oesophageal plexus
         ↙          ↘
Anterior vagal trunk      Posterior vagal trunk
       ↓  ↘   Gastric branch   ↙  ↓
       ↓        ↘             ↙   Posterior nerve of
       ↓         branch to porta  Laterjet (branches to
       ↓         hepatis          lesser curve only)
Anterior nerve of Laterjet             ↓
       ↓                          Coeliac plexus
Pylorus with branches
to lesser curve of stomach
                          along branches of coeliac axis
                          and superior mesenteric artery
                          to abdominal viscera. Ganglia
                          are found on the end organ
```

Fig. 23 The parasympathetic nervous system: cranial outflow.

```
Anterior rami of 2nd, 3rd and 4th
      sacral spinal nerves
                │
                ▼
     Pelvic splanchnic nerves
        (nervi erigentes)
                │
                ▼
        Pelvic plexus ──────────────▶ Superior hypogastric
                │                            plexus
                ▼                              │
     Inferior hypogastric                     ▼
          plexus                    Viscera along distribution
                │                     of inferior mesenteric
                ▼                            artery
        Pelvic viscera
```

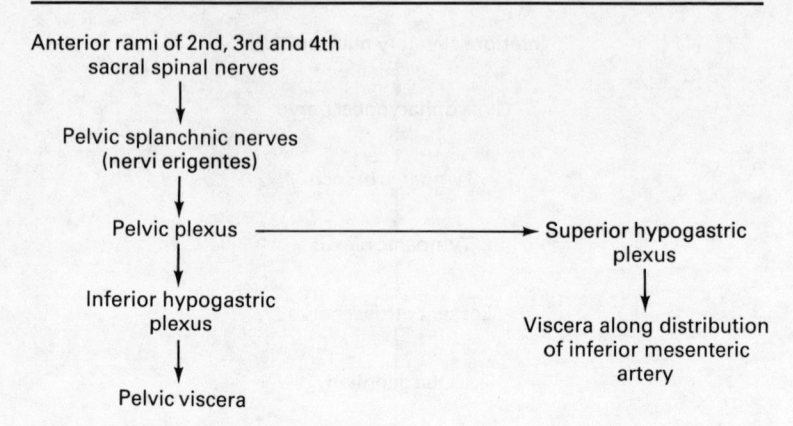

Fig. 24 Sacral parasympathetic outflow.

SPINAL CORD

The spinal cord is the caudal extension of the central nervous system which occupies the vertebral canal. It extends from the medulla oblongata to the conus medullaris, from where the filum terminale continues caudally to the coccyx.

EXTERNAL STRUCTURES

1. Meninges
   a. dura mater
   b. subdural space
   c. arachnoid mater
   d. subarachnoid space (contains cerebrospinal fluid)
   e. pia mater
2. Nerve roots
   a. anterior roots (motor and sympathetic fibres)
   b. posterior roots (sensory fibres and the spinal ganglion)
   c. they unite in the intervertebral foramen to form the spinal nerves
   d. they leave the vertebral column through the intervertebral foramina above their relevant level (C1–C7) and below their relevant level (C8 downwards)
3. Cauda equina
   The collection of nerve roots which run caudally after the spinal cord has ended between the 1st and 2nd lumbar vertebrae.

INTERNAL STRUCTURES

1. Grey columns

a. anterior horn cells (motor)
   b. posterior horn cells (sensory)
   c. lateral horn cells (sympathetic)
2. White columns
   Myelinated nerve fibres which travel up and down the spinal cord
3. Central canal
   a. runs the length of the spinal cord
   b. connects cranially with the 4th ventricle
   c. contains cerebrospinal fluid
   d. ends in the filum terminale
4. Filum terminale: the caudal extension of the pia mater after the spinal cord has terminated
5. Blood supply
   a. anterior spinal artery
   b. posterior spinal artery ($\times 2$). Both these are branches of the vertebral arteries in the cranium. These arteries descend down the spinal cord and are boosted by spinal branches from
      (i) vertebral arteries
      (ii) posterior intercostal arteries
      (iii) first lumbar arteries

RELATIONSHIP OF SPINAL CORD AND SPINAL NERVES TO THE VERTEBRAL COLUMN

1. Cervical segments: one higher than cervical vertebrae (e.g. C7 is at the level of the 6th cervical vertebra)
2. Upper thoracic segments: two higher than thoracic vertebra (e.g. T6 is at the level of the 4th thoracic vertebra)
3. Lower thoracic segments: three higher than vertebral level (e.g. L1 is at the level of the 10th thoracic vertebra)

Spinal nerves leave the vertebral column through the intervertebral foramina:
1. Spinal nerves C1–C7 leave *above* 1st to 7th cervical vertebrae
2. Spinal nerves C8 onwards leave *below* 7th cervical vertebra and onwards

Respiratory system

The respiratory system is involved in the passage of air from the mouth and nose down to the alveoli. Its origin from the primitive pharynx, which is primarily alimentary in function, explains many structural, functional, and pathological features associated with the respiratory system.

The respiratory system includes:
1. the larynx
2. the trachea
3. the principal bronchi
4. the bronchial tree
5. the lungs
6. the pleura
7. the mediastinum

The nose and mouth are described under the special senses and gastrointestinal system respectively (see p. 191 and p. 76).

LARYNX

The larynx is an organ of phonation, an air passage and a sphincter mechanism. It lies between the root of the tongue and the trachea, opposite the 3rd to 6th cervical vertebrae.

STRUCTURES

Cartilages
1. Thyroid cartilage
2. Cricoid cartilage
3. Arytenoid cartilages (×2)
4. Corniculate cartilages (×2)
5. Cuneiform cartilages (×2): lie in aryepiglottic folds
6. Epiglottis: attaches to posterior surface of thyroid cartilage in the midline, below the thyroid notch

Ligaments and membranes

Extrinsic
1. Thyrohyoid membrane

2. Median thyrohyoid ligament (middle part of thyrohyoid membrane)
3. Lateral thyrohyoid ligament
4. Hyoepiglottic ligament
5. Thyroepiglottic ligament
6. Cricotracheal ligament

Intrinsic
1. Quadrangular (quadrate) membrane
2. Cricothyroid ligament (cricovocal membrane)
3. Vocal ligaments
4. Aryepiglottic folds
5. Vestibular folds
6. Vocal folds
7. Sinus of larynx: between vestibular and vocal folds
8. Rima glottidis: fissure between the vocal folds

Intrinsic muscles
1. Thyroarytenoids ⎫ alter tension
2. Posterior cricoarytenoids ⎬ on the vocal
3. Cricothyroids ⎭ ligaments
4. Posterior cricoarytenoids: open rima glottidis
5. Lateral cricoarytenoids ⎫ close rima
6. Transverse arytenoid ⎭ glottidis
7. Oblique arytenoids ⎫ close inlet
8. Aryepiglotticus ⎭ to larynx
9. Thyroepiglotticus: widens inlet to larynx

MUCOUS MEMBRANE
Lines cavity of larynx in continuity with that of the pharynx above and the trachea below. It forms the various folds of the larynx by covering the membranes and ligaments. A few taste buds are scattered over the mucous membrane of the posterior surface of the epiglottis.

BLOOD SUPPLY
Laryngeal branches of superior and inferior thyroid arteries

VENOUS DRAINAGE
1. Superior thyroid vein
2. Inferior thyroid vein

LYMPH DRAINAGE
Deep cervical lymph nodes

NERVE SUPPLY
1. Internal branch of superior laryngeal nerve (sensory above vocal folds)
2. External branch of superior laryngeal nerve (cricothyroid muscle)
3. Recurrent laryngeal nerve, sensory below vocal folds and motor to all intrinsic muscles of the larynx except cricothyroid

TRACHEA
The trachea is a fibromuscular tube which runs from the lower border of the cricoid cartilage to its bifurcation at the carina, opposite the lower border of the 4th thoracic vertebrae. The thyroid isthmus crosses the 2nd to 4th tracheal rings.

POSITION
It lies in the lower part of the neck and the superior mediastinum anterior to the oesophagus.

STRUCTURE
Macroscopic
1. 10 cm long
2. 2 cm wide
3. Enclosed in pretracheal fascia
4. Consists of 16–20 C-shaped cartilaginous rings connected by a fibrous membrane
5. The 1st tracheal ring is attached to the cricoid cartilage by the cricotracheal ligament
6. Trachealis muscle completes the circumference of the lumen posteriorly where there is no cartilage

Microscopic
1. Respiratory epithelium (ciliated, pseudostratified)
2. Loose submucous coat with mucous glands.

BLOOD SUPPLY
Inferior thyroid artery

VENOUS DRAINAGE
Inferior thyroid vein

LYMPH DRAINAGE
1. Pretracheal lymph nodes
2. Paratracheal lymph nodes

NERVE SUPPLY
1. Sympathetic from middle cervical ganglion: bronchodilatation
2. Parasympathetic from recurrent laryngeal nerves:
   a. bronchostriction
   b. secretomotor
   c. sensory

PRINCIPAL BRONCHI
The principal bronchi run obliquely downwards and laterally to the hilum of the lung on each side.

RIGHT PRINCIPAL BRONCHUS
1. 2.5 cm long
2. Runs more vertical than left
3. Branches
   a. superior lobe bronchus
   b. middle lobe bronchus
   c. lower lobe bronchus

LEFT PRINCIPAL BRONCHUS
1. 5 cm long
2. Branches
   a. superior lobe bronchus
   b. inferior lobe bronchus

(The lingular branch is a branch from the superior lobe bronchus)

STRUCTURE
Similar to the trachea with incomplete cartilaginous rings united by a fibrous membrane.

BLOOD SUPPLY
Bronchial arteries

VENOUS DRAINAGE
Bronchial veins

LYMPH DRAINAGE
Tracheobronchial lymph nodes

NERVE SUPPLY
Autonomic supply from pulmonary plexus

BRONCHIAL TREE
The principal bronchi divide into the secondary bronchi which in turn divide into tertiary bronchi which supply the *bronchopulmonary* segments.

RIGHT LUNG
Upper lobe bronchus
1. Apical
2. Posterior
3. Anterior

Middle lobe bronchus
1. Lateral
2. Medial

Inferior lobe bronchus
1. Superior (apical)
2. Medial basal
3. Anterior basal
4. Lateral basal
5. Posterior basal

LEFT LUNG
Superior lobe
1. Apical
2. Posterior
3. Anterior
4. Superior lingular
5. Inferior lingular

Inferior lobe
1. Superior (apical)
2. Medial basal
3. Anterior basal
4. Lateral basal
5. Posterior basal

FURTHER DIVISIONS

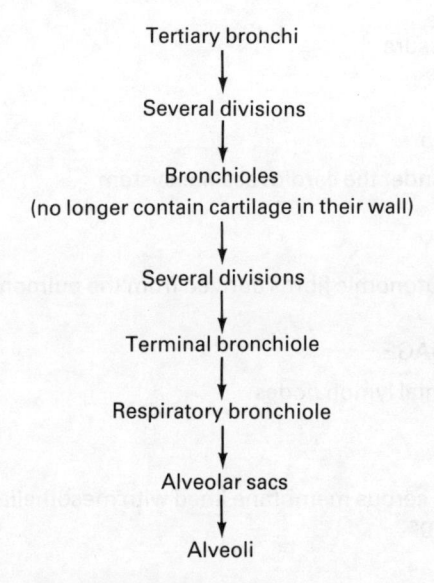

```
Tertiary bronchi
       ↓
Several divisions
       ↓
   Bronchioles
(no longer contain cartilage in their wall)
       ↓
Several divisions
       ↓
Terminal bronchiole
       ↓
Respiratory bronchiole
       ↓
  Alveolar sacs
       ↓
     Alveoli
```

Fig. 25 Further divisions of the bronchial tree.

The mucous membrane alters from respiratory epithelium to non-ciliated cuboidal epithelium in the smaller bronchioles. Finally, the alveolar ducts, sacs and alveoli are lined with simple squamous cells. The elastic framework of this system provides the elastic recoil of the lungs during expiration.

LUNGS

The lung are the organs of respiration, occupying both pleural cavities and are separated from each other by the contents of the mediastinum.

RIGHT LUNG

1. Upper lobe
2. Horizontal fissure
3. Middle lobe
4. Oblique fissure
5. Lower lobe

LEFT LUNG

1. Upper lobe
2. Oblique fissure
3. Lower lobe

BLOOD SUPPLY

As described under the cardiovascular system

NERVE SUPPLY

Comes from autonomic fibres derived from the pulmonary plexus

LYMPH DRAINAGE

Tracheobronchial lymph nodes

PLEURA

The pleura is a serous membrane lined with mesothelial cells which invests the lungs.

STRUCTURE

1. Parietal layer
2. Visceral layer
3. Pulmonary ligaments: the double layer of pleura below the hilum of each lung

BLOOD AND NERVE SUPPLY

1. Parietal pleura: vessels and nerves of the body wall
2. Visceral pleura: bronchial vessels and nerves

MEDIASTINUM

The mediastinum is the partition between the two lungs. For descriptive purposes it is divided into upper and lower compartments.

UPPER (SUPERIOR) MEDIASTINUM

Boundaries
1. Above line from manubrium to 4th thoracic vertebrae
2. Below line from manubrium to 1st thoracic vertebrae

Contents
1. Aortic arch and its branches

2. Brachiocephalic veins and upper half of superior vena cava
3. Left superior intercostal vein
4. Vagus nerves
5. Phrenic nerves
6. Left recurrent laryngeal nerve
7. Trachea
8. Oesophagus
9. Thoracic duct
10. Thymus
11. Lymph nodes

LOWER MEDIASTINUM
Boundaries
1. Below superior mediastinum
2. Behind sternum
3. In front of vertebral column
4. Between the lungs

Contents
Anterior mediastinum (between sternum and pericardium)
1. Lymph nodes
2. Branches of internal thoracic artery

Middle mediastinum
1. Heart
2. Pericardium
3. Ascending aorta
4. Lower part of superior vena cava
5. Azygos vein
6. Bifurcation of trachea
7. Main bronchi
8. Pulmonary trunk
9. Pulmonary veins
10. Phrenic nerves
11. Cardiac plexus
12. Lymph nodes

Posterior mediastinum (behind middle mediastinum)
1. Descending thoracic aorta
2. Azygos vein
3. Hemiazygos vein
4. Vagus nerves
5. Splanchnic nerves
6. Oesophagus
7. Thoracic duct
8. Lymph nodes

Gastrointestinal system

The gastrointestinal system extends from the mouth to the anus and comprises the alimentary tract with its accessory organs. Apart from most of the oesophagus and the anal canal, the gastrointestinal tract lies wholly within the abdominal cavity.

MOUTH
The mouth extends from the lips and cheeks backwards to the palatoglossal arch (anterior pillar of fauces). It is divided by the gums into the vestibule and the oral cavity. The roof of the mouth is formed by the palate, with mylohyoid muscle and the tongue forming the floor.

PARTS
1. Vestibule
   a. opening of parotid duct (opposite upper 2nd molar teeth)
   b. openings of many smaller solitary glands
2. Oral cavity
   a. frenulum linguae
   b. sublingual papillae: with the openings of the submandibular ducts on each side
3. Teeth
   a. enamel
   b. dentine
   c. pulp
4. Palate
   a. hard palate
      (i) palatine processes of maxillae
      (ii) horizontal plates of palatine bones
   b. soft palate
      (i) aponeurosis
      (ii) uvula
   c. palatine musculature
      (i) levator veli palatini
      (ii) tensor veli palatini

          (iii) palatoglossus (anterior pillar of fauces)
          (iv) palatopharyngeus (posterior pillar of fauces)
   5. Tongue
      a. intrinsic muscles
          (i) superior and inferior longitudinal fibres
          (ii) transverse fibres
          (iii) vertical fibres
      b. extrinsic muscles
          (i) genioglossus (body of tongue)
          (ii) hyoglossus
          (iii) styloglossus
      c. median fibrous septum: divides the tongue into two halves
      d. Foramen caecum
      e. Sulcus terminalis: separates posterior one-third from anterior two-thirds
      f. Papillae
          (i) vallatae
          (ii) fungiform
          (iii) filiform

STRUCTURE

A *mucous membrane* of stratified squamous epithelium covers the inside of the mouth, forming the gingiva around the insertion of the teeth. It contains numerous mucous glands. The tongue contains papillae over the anterior two-thirds which increase the surface of the mucous membrane coming into contact with the substance being tasted.

Taste buds are the peripheral gustatory organs and are formed in the epithelium covering the tongue, inferior surface of soft palate, palatoglossal arches, posterior surface of epiglottis, and posterior wall of the oropharynx.

ARTERIAL SUPPLY

1. From maxillary artery
   a. inferior alveolar artery
   b. posterior superior alveolar artery
   c. infraorbital artery (anterior superior alveolar branch)
   d. greater palatine artery
2. From ascending pharyngeal artery: pharyngeal branch (to palate)
3. From lingual artery
   a. dorsal lingual artery
   b. sublingual artery
4. From facial artery
   a. ascending palatine artery
   b. submental artery

c. inferior labial artery
   d. superior labial artery

VENOUS DRAINAGE
1. Pterygoid plexus
2. Maxillary vein
3. Facial vein
4. Tonsillar plexus

LYMPH DRAINAGE
1. Superior deep cervical lymph nodes (Jugulodigastric node: tonsil)
2. Inferior deep cervical lymph nodes (Jugulo-omohyoid node: tongue)

NERVE SUPPLY
Sensory
1. From maxillary nerve
   a. anterior palatine nerve
   b. nasopalatine nerve
   c. anterior superior alveolar nerve
   d. middle superior alveolar nerve
   e. posterior superior alveolar nerve
   f. greater palatine nerve
   g. lesser palatine nerve
2. From mandibular nerve
   a. inferior alveolar nerve
   b. lingual nerve
   c. buccal nerve

Taste
1. From lingual nerve: fibres run to chorda tympani then to nervus intermedius (from anterior two-thirds of tongue)
2. From glossopharyngeal nerve: taste from pharyngeal part of tongue (posterior one-third)

Motor
1. From hypoglossal nerve: to muscles of tongue
2. From vagus nerve: carrying fibres from cranial part of accessory nerve to pharyngeal plexus
3. From mandibular nerve: from branch to medial pterygoid muscle which supplies tensor veli palatini

SALIVARY GLANDS

The salivary glands comprise three main paired glands (parotid, submandibular, sublingual), the anterior lingual glands, and numerous small glands in the mucous membrane of the lips, cheek and palate. They secrete saliva which can be serous or mucoid. Each salivary gland consists of lobes, which are made up of lobules and which, in turn, are formed by a single duct draining several alveoli.

PAROTID GLAND

Position
1. Below the external auditory meatus
2. Between the mandible and sternocleidomastoid
3. Extends anteriorly over masseter

Structure
Macroscopic
1. Capsule: deep cervical fascia
2. Superficial part
3. Deep part
4. Parotid duct: opens through cheek opposite upper 2nd molar teeth

Microscopic
Serous alveoli: structures within the gland include
1. External carotid artery (Deep part of gland)
2. Maxillary artery
3. Superficial temporal artery
4. Retromandibular vein
5. Branches of facial nerve (superficial part of gland)

Vascular supply
1. Branches of external carotid artery
2. Venous drainage to external jugular vein

Lymph drainage
1. Superficial cervical lymph nodes
2. Deep cervical lymph nodes (via lymph nodes on the surface of the gland itself)

Nerve supply
1. Auriculo-temporal nerve: secretomotor (parasympathetic fibres from tympanic branch of glossopharyngeal nerve via otic ganglion)
2. Sympathetic vasoconstrictor fibres (from carotid plexus)

SUBMANDIBULAR GLAND

Position
1. Under mandible
2. Superficial part
   a. lateral to mylohyoid
   b. medial to mandibular branch of facial nerve
   c. lateral to digastric tendon
3. Deep part: between mylohyoid (lateral) and hyoglossus (medial)

Structure

Macroscopic
1. Covered on its external surface by the deep cervical fascia
2. Submandibular duct: opens on each side of frenulum in the floor of the mouth

Microscopic
Serous and mucous alveoli (mainly serous)

Vascular supply
1. Branches of
   a. facial artery
   b. lingual artery
2. Venous drainage follows course of arteries

Lymph drainage
Submandibular lymph nodes

Nerve supply
1. Parasympathetic secretomotor fibres from the chorda tympani (branch of facial nerve) run to the submandibular ganglion in the lingual nerve
2. Sympathetic vasoconstrictor fibres run to the submandibular gland along the arteries.

SUBLINGUAL GLAND

Position
1. Under mucous membrane of floor of mouth
2. In the sublingual fossa of mandible, near the symphysis

Structure

Macroscopic
Sublingual salivary ducts open into floor of mouth

Microscopic
Serous and mucous alveoli (mainly mucous)

Gastrointestinal system

Vascular supply
1. Sublingual artery and vein
2. Submental artery and vein

Lymph drainage
Submental lymph nodes

Nerve supply
Same as for the submandibular gland

PHARYNX

The pharynx is a musculomembraneous tube which lies behind the nasal cavities, mouth and larynx. It extends from the base of the skull to the commencement of the oesophagus, at the lower border of the cricoid cartilage, level with the 6th cervical vertebrae.
 It is divided into three anatomical parts:
1. Nasopharynx
2. Oropharynx
3. Laryngeal part

WALL

1. Pharyngobasilar fascia
2. Superior constrictor
   a. origin
      (i) medial pterygoid plate
      (ii) pterygomandibular raphé
   b. insertion
      (i) pharyngeal tubercle
      (ii) median pharyngeal raphé
3. Middle constrictor
   a. origin
      (i) stylohyoid ligament
      (ii) hyoid bone
   b. insertion: median raphé
4. Inferior constrictor consists of two parts:
   Thyropharyngeus
   a. origin: oblique line of thyroid cartilage
   b. insertion: median raphé
   Cricopharyngeus
   Extends from one cricoid arch to the other, acting as a sphincter to the upper end of the oesophagus

MUSCLES ACTING ON PHARYNX

1. Stylopharyngeus (glossopharyngeal nerve)
2. Salpingopharyngeus (pharyngeal plexus)

3. Stylohyoid (facial nerve)
4. Passavant's muscle: part of palatopharyngeus which encircles the pharynx within the superior constrictor (pharyngeal plexus)

PARTS AND STRUCTURES

Nasopharynx

Position
Above soft palate, behind nasal cavities

Structures
1. Pharyngeal opening of auditory tube
2. Salpingopharyngeal fold
3. Salpingopalatine fold
4. Pharyngeal recess
5. Pharyngeal tonsils
6. Tubal tonsils

Sensory nerve supply
Maxillary nerve (branches of pterygopalatine ganglion)

Oropharynx

Position
Between soft palate and upper border of epiglottis

Structures
1. Palatopharyngeal arch (Posterior pillar of fauces or palatopharyngeus)
2. Palatine tonsils

Sensory nerve supply
1. Glossopharyngeal nerve
2. Maxillary nerve (palatine branches)

Laryngeal part of pharynx

Position
Below cranial border of epiglottis

Structures
1. Laryngeal orifice
2. Piriform fossae (on each side of laryngeal orifice)

Sensory nerve supply
Vagus nerve (from internal laryngeal nerves)

STRUCTURE

Microscopic
1. Mucous membrane
   a. ciliated columnar (nasopharynx)
   b. stratified squamous (oral and laryngeal parts)
2. Fibrous layer
   a. between mucosa and muscular layer
   b. strengthened superiorly as pharyngobasilar fascia and posteriorly as the median pharyngeal raphé
3. Muscle layer: constrictors of pharynx

ARTERIAL SUPPLY

1. Ascending pharyngeal artery
2. Ascending palatine artery
3. Tonsillar branch of facial artery
4. Greater palatine artery ⎫
5. Pharyngeal artery   ⎬ branches of maxillary artery
6. Artery of pterygoid canal ⎭
7. Dorsal lingual branches of lingual artery

VENOUS DRAINAGE

Through a venous plexus which drains into the internal jugular and facial veins. It communicates above with the pterygoid plexus

NERVE SUPPLY

Sensory
1. Maxillary nerve
2. Glossopharyngeal nerve

Motor
Cranial part of the accessory nerve which reaches the pharyngeal plexus via the Vagus nerve; supplies all muscles of pharynx except:
1. Stylopharyngeus (IX)
2. Tensor veli palatini (mandibular nerve)

Autonomic

Parasympathetic
1. Glossopharyngeal nerve
2. Vagus nerve

Sympathetic
Superior cervical ganglion
The nerve fibres to the pharynx are distributed via the pharyngeal

plexus which lies in the connective tissue external to the pharyngeal constrictors.

LYMPH DRAINAGE

Retropharyngeal nodes to the upper deep cervical nodes

Special group of pharyngeal lymph nodes

Waldeyer's ring
A ring of lymphoid tissue which surrounds the upper part of the pharynx. Its components are shown in Figure 25.

```
                    Pharyngeal tonsil (adenoids)
Tubal nodes                                              Tubal nodes

Palatine tonsil                                          Palatine tonsil
                         Lingual tonsil
```

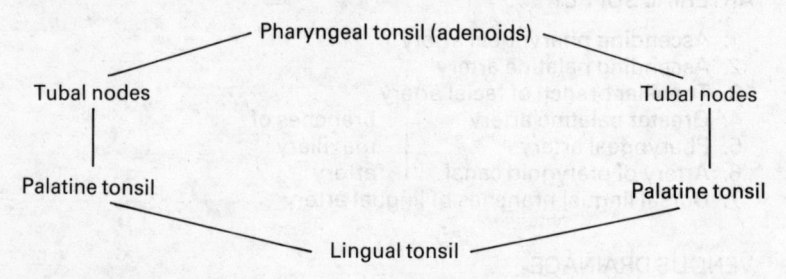

Fig. 26 Waldeyer's ring.

Palatine tonsil: the largest of these components
1. Blood supply
   a. tonsillar branch of facial artery
   b. ascending palatine branch of facial artery
   c. dorsal lingual branches of lingual artery
   d. greater palatine branch of maxillary artery
2. Venous drainage
   a. external palatine vein
   b. pharyngeal vein
   c. facial vein
3. Nerve supply: from pterygopalatine ganglion and glossopharyngeal nerve
4. Lymphatic drainage: jugulodigastric node

OESOPHAGUS

The oesophagus is a muscular tube, approximately 25 cm long, which extends from the cricoid cartilage and cricopharyngeus proximally, to the cardiac orifice of the stomach. There are four places in its course where the oesophagus is constricted:
1. At the commencement at cricopharyngeus
2. Where it is crossed by the aortic arch

Gastrointestinal system

3. Where it is crossed by the left main bronchus
4. Where it pierces the diaphragm

PARTS

Cervical part
1. Lies behind trachea
2. Recurrent laryngeal nerves lie lateral
3. Lies on the pre-vertebral muscles

Thoracic part
1. Runs from superior mediastinum through the posterior mediastinum to the diaphragm
2. It is related in its course to the left atrium
3. The vagus nerves descend in close contact with the oesophagus
4. Lies anterior to the descending aorta

Abdominal part
1. Emerges from right crus of diaphragm at the level of the 10th thoracic vertebrae
2. It is between 1–2 cm long
3. Its right border continues into the lesser curve of the stomach

STRUCTURE

Microscopic
Mucous membrane: stratified squamous epithelium
1. Submucosa: contains mucous glands, vessels and nerves
2. Muscular layer
   a. inner circular
   b. outer longitudinal
3. External fibrous layer (only the intra-abdominal part is covered with serosa)

ARTERIAL SUPPLY

1. Inferior thyroid artery
2. Branches from descending aorta
3. Bronchial arteries
4. Left gastric artery
5. Left inferior phrenic artery

VENOUS DRAINAGE

1. Inferior thyroid veins
2. Azygos vein
3. Hemiazygos vein

4. Accessory hemiazygos vein
5. Left gastric vein

LYMPH DRAINAGE

Paratracheal lymph nodes
Posterior mediastinal nodes

NERVE SUPPLY

Parasympathetic
1. Motor
2. Secretomotor } vagus nerve

Sympathetic
Vasomotor: middle and inferior cervical and upper thoracic ganglia

STOMACH

The stomach is the widest and most distensible part of the alimentary canal. It lies in the left upper quadrant of the abdomen, forming a J-shape (although the shape and position may vary considerably).

POSITION

Lies between the cardia, situated just below the oesophageal opening in the diaphragm at the level of T10, behind the 7th costal cartilage 2 cm to the left of the midline, and the pylorus at the level of L1. The stomach lies on the stomach bed.

Stomach bed (from above-down)
1. Diaphragm
2. Spleen
3. Left adrenal
4. Left kidney
5. Splenic artery
6. Pancreas
7. Transverse mesocolon and colon

STRUCTURE

Macroscopic
1. Cardia
2. Greater curvature
3. Lesser curvature
4. Fundus
5. Body and antrum

Gastrointestinal system

6. Pylorus
7. Incisura angularis (constant notch two-thirds down lesser curve)

Microscopic
From outside inwards:
1. Serosa: formed by the peritoneum which encloses the whole surface of the stomach except for a small bare area to the left of the cardia
2. Muscularis externa: three layers
   a. outer longitudinal
   b. inner circular which is thickened at the pylorus to form a sphincter
   c. innermost oblique limited to the body of the stomach
3. Submucosa: loose areolar tissue containing vessels and nerves
4. Mucosa: thrown into folds called rugae which consist of
   a. columnar secretory epithelium producing mucus
   b. gastric glands opening into gastric pits comprising:
      (i) cardiac glands which secrete mucus
      (ii) main gastric glands of the body and fundus have four cell types:
         — chief cells: secrete pepsin
         — oxyntic (parietal): secrete acid
         — mucous neck cells: secrete mucus
         — argentaffin cells
      (iii) Pyloric glands which secrete gastrin
   c. lymphatic follicles lie amongst the glands
   d. muscularis mucosa lies deep to the glands

BLOOD SUPPLY

1. Left gastric artery
2. Right gastric artery
3. Right gastroepiploic artery
4. Left gastroepiploic artery
5. Short gastric arteries (four to five in number)

VENOUS DRAINAGE

1. Left gastric vein ⎫
2. Right gastric vein ⎬ drain into portal vein
3. Prepyloric veins ⎭
4. Left gastroepiploic vein ⎫ drain into
5. Short gastric veins ⎭ the splenic vein
6. Right gastroepiploic vein: drains into the superior mesenteric vein

NERVE SUPPLY

Parasympthetic
These are motor and secretomotor from the vagus nerve.
1. The anterior vagus (left vagal fibres) via
   a. cardiac branches
   b. gastric branches from the greater anterior gastric nerve which runs along lesser curve in the lesser omentum
   c. pyloric branches
2. The posterior vagus (right vagal fibres) via
   a. gastric branches from the greater posterior gastric nerve lying along posterior margin of the lesser curve
   b. coeliac branches to coeliac plexus

Sympathetic
Via the coeliac plexus and some fibres from the hepatic plexus, inferior phrenic plexus and direct from splanchnic nerves. These are vasomotor, inhibitory to muscle and sensory.

LYMPHATIC DRAINAGE

Accompanying vessels to:
1. Left gastric nodes from both surfaces of stomach
2. Pancreaticosplenic nodes: drain fundus and body of stomach on the left side
3. Right gastro-epiploic nodes from greater curvature
4. Pyloric and hepatic nodes: drain the pyloric region

All ultimately pass to the coeliac pre-aortic nodes.

SMALL INTESTINE

This extends from the pylorus to the ileocaecal valve. Approximately 5 m in length in the living state, it comprises three parts:
1. Duodenum
2. Jejunum
3. Ileum

DUODENUM

The duodenum encloses the head of the pancreas in a C-shape running from the pylorus to the duodenojejunal flexure. It receives the secretions of the biliary and pancreatic systems.
25 cm in length, it is the shortest part of the intestine.

Position
The upper limb of the C-shape runs from the pylorus at the level of L1 to cross aorta and IVC. It then runs in right para-aortic gutter down to the level of L3, crosses major vessels again to end at the

duodenojejunal flexure, 2.5 cm to the left of the midline and 1 cm below transpyloric plane.

Structure

Macroscopic
This comprises four parts
   1st part (superior): 5 cm long. Pylorus to neck of gallbladder. Invested with peritoneum completely except posteriorly.
   2nd part (descending): 10 cm long. Neck of gallbladder to level of L3. Covered anteriorly by peritoneum except where the transverse colon crosses it. Posteromedial wall has the major duodenal papilla (8–10 cm distal to pylorus), the opening of the common bile duct and pancreatic duct conjoined as the ampulla. Minor duodenal papilla lies 2 cm proximal to the major papilla and is the opening of the accessory pancreatic duct.
   3rd part (horizontal): 10 cm long. Right side of aorta to left para-aortic gutter at the level of L3. Covered anteriorly by peritoneum except where superior mesenteric vessels cross.
   4th part (ascending): 2.5 cm. Left para-aortic gutter to the duodenojejunal flexure at the level of L2. Covered by peritoneum anteriorly. Supported by the muscle of Trietz: striated and smooth muscle originating from the right crus of diaphragm attaching to duodenojejunal flexure. Peritoneal folds form the paraduodenal fossae at the duodenojejunal flexure:
1. Paraduodenal
2. Retroduodenal
3. Superior duodenal
4. Inferior duodenal

Blood supply
1. Right gastric artery
2. Supraduodenal artery
3. Right gastroepiploic
4. Superior and inferior pancreaticoduodenal arteries
5. Hepatic artery

Venous Drainage
Corresponding veins into
1. Splenic vein
2. Superior mesenteric vein
3. Portal vein

Lymphatic Drainage
Accompany arteries to end in:
1. Hepatic nodes
2. Coeliac nodes
3. Superior mesenteric nodes

Nerve supply
Autonomic: sympathetic and parasympathetic from the coeliac plexus. Accompanying arterial supply.

JEJUNUM & ILEUM
Position
Average length is 5 m. Division between jejunum and ileum is arbitrary. Approximate guide:
1. Upper two-fifths: jejunum
2. Lower three-fifths: ileum
   Extends from duodenojejunal flexure to ileocaecal valve.

Completely invested with peritoneum, lying free in coils within the abdominal cavity. Attached to posterior abdominal wall by the mesentery.

Structure
Macroscopic
Luminal aspect of small intestine thrown into folds called plicae circulares; crescenteric folds of mucous membrane which begins 2–5 cm distal to the pylorus where they are large and numerous, at the mid-ileum they have almost disappeared.

Jejunum
1. 4 cm diameter
2. Thick walled, vascular, circular folds are thicker than in the ileum

Ileum
1. 3.5 cm diameter
2. Thin-walled
3. Circular folds of mucous membrane disappear towards terminal part
4. Aggregated lymphatic follicles (Peyer's patches)
5. Meckel's diverticulum (60 cm proximal to ileocaecal valve; 5 cm long; in 2% of the population) is the persisting remnant of the vitelline duct

Blood supply
Superior mesenteric artery: jejunal and ileal branches and ileocolic artery to the terminal part of ileum.

Venous drainage
Corresponding veins into the superior mesenteric vein

Lymphatic drainage
Lymphatic plexuses in the gut wall run to mesenteric and ileocolic nodes to superior mesenteric pre-aortic nodes. Accompany arteries.

Nerve supply

Autonomic
1. Sympathetic: splanchnic nerves via the coeliac plexus along the arterial supply
2. Parasympathetic: vagus nerve

Nerves are distributed in Meissner (submucosal) and Auerbach's (myenteric) plexuses in the gut wall.

Sympathetic
Vasomotor; inhibitory to peristalsis and contracts sphincters

Parasympathetic
1. Motor to muscle
2. Relaxes sphincters
3. Secretomotor

Structure

Microscopic
1. Serous layer: visceral peritoneum
2. Muscularis externa (smooth muscle)
   a. outer fibres longitudinal
   b. inner fibres circular
3. Submucous layer: loose connective tissue which contains blood vessels lymphatics and nerves
4. Mucous membrane: consists of three layers:
   a. muscularis mucosa:
      (i) outer longitudinal fibres
      (ii) inner circular fibres
   b. lamina propria
   c. basement membrane: supporting a columnar epithelium

Villi
1. Finger-like projections from mucous membrane which increase the surface area of the gut
2. Thin and tall in jejunum, broader and shorter in ileum
3. Consists of a core of reticular tissue containing lacteal, vessels and smooth muscle
4. Lined by columnar absorptive epithelium with a few goblet cells

Glands
1. Duodenum: mucous tubulo-alveolar glands called Brunners glands, extend through the muscularis mucosa into the submucous layer
2. Intestinal (Crypts of Lieberkuhn):
   a. extend into the mucosa between villi
   b. consists of simple tubular glands

Cells lining the glands are:
1. Columnar epithelial cells which migrate upwards from base of gland
2. Paneth cells: produce digestive enzymes
3. Argentaffin cells: part of APUD system. Derived from neural crest

Scattered throughout mucous membrane of the small intestine are solitary lymphatic follicles. These are densely populated areas of lymphocytes and towards the ileum they form large aggregated follicles known as Peyers patches (10–260 follicles, 2–10 cm in length).

LARGE INTESTINE

The large intestine extends from ileum to anus and is 1.5 m long. Its calibre is widest at caecum, gradually diminishing until the rectum. Unlike the small intestine, it is more fixed in position and acts to absorb fluid and electrolytes.

POSITION

Starts at caecum in right iliac fossa and ascends to right hypochondrium just below transpyloric plane. Swings across midline to left hypochondrium just above transpyloric plane. Descends to pelvic inlet and after a sigmoid loop continues in the midline on the sacrum to the anal canal.

PARTS

Caecum
1. 6 × 7.5 cm in length and breadth
2. Lies in right iliac fossa superior to lateral half of inguinal ligament
3. Base of appendix joins posteromedial wall, 2 cm below ileocaecal valve which enters at the junction of ascending colon and caecum.

Appendix
1. Base marked by McBurney's point on abdominal wall
2. 2–20 cm in length

Position
1. Retrocaecal: 65%
2. Pelvic: 31%
3. Subcaecal: 2.26%
4. Preileal: 1%
5. Postileal: 0.4%
6. Connected to terminal ileum by meso-appendix

Gastrointestinal system

Ascending colon
1. 15 cm in length
2. Fixed down by peritoneum in right colic gutter. Ends at the right colic flexure

Transverse colon
1. 50 cm in length
2. Lies free invested by peritoneum and attached via transverse mesocolon
3. Forms a convex loop downwards: position may vary, considerably
4. Ends at the left colic flexure

Descending colon
1. 25 cm in length
2. Fixed down by peritoneum in left colic gutter

Sigmoid colon
1. 40 cm long
2. Lies free on the sigmoid mesocolon
3. Lies in pelvis and is usually mobile

Rectum
1. 12 cm long
2. Anteroposterior curve follows the curve of the sacrum
3. Three lateral curves form three constant horizontal folds called valves of Houston:
   a. upper: convex to the right
   b. middle: convex to left
   c. lower: convex to right; dilated as rectal ampulla.

Peritoneal covering of the rectum
1. Upper one-third: front and sides
2. Middle one-third: front only
Peritoneum is reflected upwards to form
1. Rectovesical pouch in men
2. Recto-uterine pouch in women

STRUCTURE

Microscopic
Layers similar to those of small intestine.

Serosa
Visceral peritoneum with peritoneal pouches filled with fat, called the *appendices epiploica*. These cover the surface of the colon. Absent on the rectum.

Muscularis Externa
1. Outer longitudinal layer is a continuous circumferential layer. Thickened to form three longitudinal bundles, the *taeniae coli*. 6–12 mm wide. Start at the base of appendix and extend to sigmoid colon
2. Taeniae are shorter than other layers and cause the colon to produce its characteristic sacculated appearance (haustrations)
3. Inner circular layer of muscle is continuous throughout the whole length

Submucous layer
Loose connective tissue containing vessels, lymphatics and nerves

Mucous membrane
1. Muscularis mucosa
   a. outer longitudinal layer
   b. inner circular layer
2. Glands: tubular; lined by mucous secreting cells
3. Epithelium: columnar absorptive cells and scattered goblet cells
Solitary lymphatic follicles are numerous in appendix and caecum, and are scattered throughout large intestine.

ARTERIAL SUPPLY

The branches of the superior mesenteric artery to large intestine derived from the midgut: caecum, appendix, ascending and right two-thirds of transverse colon. Branches of inferior mesenteric artery to large intestine derived from hindgut: Left one-third of transverse, descending and sigmoid colon and rectum. Rectum also receives arterial supply from other sources.

Caecum
Anterior and posterior caecal artery ⎫
⎪
Appendix ⎪
Appendicular artery ⎬ branches of the ileocolic artery
⎪
Ascending colon ⎪
1. Ascending colic artery ⎪
2. Superior branch of ileocolic ⎪
3. Right colic artery ⎭

Transverse colon
1. Middle colic artery (right and left divisions)
2. Ascending branch of left colic artery

Descending colon
Left colic artery (ascending and descending branches)

Gastrointestinal system

Sigmoid colon
Two to three sigmoid arteries

Rectum
1. Superior rectal artery: branch of inferior mesenteric artery
2. Middle rectal artery: branch of internal iliac artery
3. Inferior rectal artery: branch of pudendal artery

Marginal artery
A single trunk running from caecum to rectum lying 1 cm from gut wall on its convex border. Formed by anastomoses between vessels described above.

VENOUS DRAINAGE

1. Correspondingly-named veins:
   a. caecum
   b. ascending colon
   c. right two-thirds of transverse colon
   d. appendix
   } to superior mesenteric vein

   e. left one-third of transverse colon
   f. descending colon
   g. sigmoid colon
   } to inferior mesenteric vein
2. Rectum is the site of portosystemic venous junctions
   a. Internal rectal plexus lies in the submucosa and drains to superior rectal vein to inferior mesenteric vein (portal system)
   b. External rectal plexus lies outside the external muscle coat and drains to middle rectal vein to internal iliac vein (systemic system)

   There is free communication between the two plexi.

LYMPHATIC DRAINAGE

Accompanies arteries

Colon
Colon has four groups of nodes
1. Epicolic: on the gut wall
2. Paracolic: along convex border of colon
3. Intermediate: along right middle and left colic arteries
4. Terminal: near main pre-aortic groups

ultimately drain into two pre-aortic groups:
— inferior mesenteric group
— superior mesenteric group

Rectum
1. Upper half drains with the superior rectal artery to inferior mesenteric group
2. Lower half with middle rectal artery to internal iliac nodes

NERVE SUPPLY

Autonomic
Distributed via Meissner's and Auerbach's plexuses in the gut wall. Nerves run with arterial supply.

Sympathetic
From splanchnic nerves via coeliac and superior mesenteric ganglia to derivatives of the midgut. From the lumbar trunk and superior hypogastric plexus to derivatives of the hindgut.

Parasympathetic
From the vagi through the coeliac plexus to the midgut. From the pelvic splanchnic nerves (nervi erigentes) to the hindgut via inferior hypogastric plexus, with some fibres passing directly to the colon on the posterior abdominal wall.

ANAL CANAL

4 cm long. Passes downwards and backwards from the anorectal junction. Anterior wall is shorter than posterior. Upper two-thirds derived from endoderm and lower one-third from ectoderm, this accounts for the division of the blood supply, lymphatic drainage and nerve supply.

STRUCTURE

Macroscopic

Anal columns
Vertical folds of mucous membrane: three enlarged
1. Left lateral ⎫ form 1°
2. Right posterior ⎬ internal
3. Right anterior ⎭ haemorrhoids

Anal valves
Crescenteric transverse folds at lower end of columns which lie along the pectinate line. This is the junction of the endodermal and ectodermal origin of the anal canal.

Anal sinuses
Small depressions above valves.

Anal papillae
Projections of mucous membrane from anal valves.

Transitional zone
Lies between pectinate line and white line of Hilton.

Gastrointestinal system 97

White line of Hilton
Lies at the lower level of the internal sphincter, forming the intersphincteric groove. Below the line the anal canal is lined by skin that contains sweat and sebaceous glands.

Anal glands
Secretory, straight and branched. Lined by stratified columnar epithelium. Open into anal crypts small depressions in region of anal sinuses. Extend into submucosa and internal sphincter.

Microscopic
1. Above pectinate line: similar to large bowel
2. Between pectinate line and white line of Hilton: transitional stratified epithelium
3. Below white line: stratified squamous epithelium, i.e. skin and its appendages

ARTERIAL SUPPLY
1. Superior rectal artery: above anal valves
2. Inferior rectal artery: below anal valves

VENOUS DRAINAGE
1. Above valves via external rectal plexus, thence to middle and superior rectal veins
2. Below valves by a rich plexus to the inferior rectal veins
   Little communication across valves

LYMPHATIC DRAINAGE

Accompany arteries
1. Above valves to pararectal nodes to inferior mesenteric nodes
2. Below valves to internal and superficial inguinal nodes

NERVE SUPPLY

Above valves
1. Autonomic via inferior and superior hypogastric plexuses
2. Parasympathetic is motor to rectum and inhibitory to internal sphincter
3. Sympathetic contracts the internal sphincter

Below valves
Somatic via the inferior rectal branch of pudendal nerve (S2, S3) and perineal branch of S4

ANAL MUSCULATURE

Circular smooth muscle of rectum thickens at the anorectal junction to form the sphincter ani internus which surrounds the upper three-quarters of the anal canal. Ends at white line of Hilton.
 Sphincter ani externus: striated muscle comprised of three parts.

Subcutaneous
1. 5 cm wide
2. Lies below internal sphincter and superficial part of external sphincter. Surrounds the anal canal
3. A few fibres are attached anteriorly to perineal body and posteriorly to anococcygeal ligament
4. Lies beneath skin

Superficial
1. Elliptical
2. Deep to subcutaneous part
3. Attached posteriorly to tip of coccyx and anococcygeal raphe
4. Inserted anteriorly to perineal body

Deep
1. Annular band which surrounds upper part of internal sphincter
2. Deep fibres fused with puborectalis

Nerve supply
Sphincter ani internus
1. Autonomic via hypogastric plexuses
    Sympathetic: contraction
    Parasympathetic: relaxation

Sphincter ani externus
1. Somatic: inferior rectal branch of pudendal nerve (S2, 3)
            perineal branch of 4th sacral nerve

LIVER

The liver is the largest organ in the body. It is wedge-shaped, occupying the right hypochondrium, part of the epigastrium and left hypochondrium. It weighs 1.0–2.5 kg and is reddish brown in colour. It has many metabolic functions and is a part of the reticulo-endothelial system.

Gastrointestinal system 99

POSITION

Surface markings

Upper border
Lies on a line connecting the xiphisternum to just below the right and left nipples.

Right border
Below right nipple to 1 cm below coastal margin at 10th costal cartilage, convex to the right.

Inferior border
Lies between lowest point of right border and left upper border, passing through the transpyloric plane.
 The liver is completely invested by peritoneum except for the bare area on the posterior surface of the right lobe.

Peritoneal connections
1. Falciform ligament
2. Coronary ligament
3. Left and right triangular ligaments
4. Lesser omentum
5. Hepatorenal ligament

STRUCTURE

Macroscopic

Lobes
The right lobe is separated from the left by fissures for the ligamentum venosum and the ligamentum teres:
1. Right
2. Left
3. Caudate ⎫ arise from
4. Quadrate ⎭ the right lobe

It is also divided segmentally according to major division of hepatic artery, portal vein and bile ducts.

Segments
1. Right lobe
   a. anterior
   b. posterior
2. Left lobe
   a. medial
   b. lateral

these segments can each be divided into superior and inferior parts

Hepatic veins lie in intersegmental positions.

Porta hepatis
The porta hepatis is situated on the inferior surface between the quadrate lobe in front and caudate lobe behind.

Contents of porta hepatis:
1. Portal vein
2. Hepatic artery
3. Hepatic ducts (right and left)
4. Lymph nodes
5. Hepatic plexus of nerves

Microscopic
1. Outer layer: thin capsule (Glissons capsule)
2. Internal architecture:
    a. hepatic lobules which are a polyhedral shape with a central vein at the centre and portal triads at the edge.
    b. Portal triad consists of the tributaries of portal vein, hepatic artery and bile duct
    c. Portal lobule is a triangle formed by joining three central veins with portal triad at the centre.
3. Cellular structure (hepatic laminae)
    a. hepatocytes which lie in sheets
    b. hepatic macrophages (Kuppfer cells) are part of the endothelial lining of intrahepatic sinusoids. Sinusoids run between hepatic sheets from portal vein to central vein. Bile canuliculi surround surfaces of cells and drain to bile in portal triads

BLOOD SUPPLY
1. Hepatic artery
2. Portal vein

VENOUS DRAINAGE
Hepatic veins direct to inferior vena cava

LYMPHATIC DRAINAGE
Superficial system
1. To nodes around inferior vena cava
2. Direct to thoracic duct
3. Nodes in porta hepatis
4. Coeliac nodes
5. Paracardial nodes through the oesophageal hiatus

Deep system
1. IVC nodes
2. Porta hepatis nodes

NERVE SUPPLY
1. Parasympathetic from vagus
2. Sympathetic from coeliac ganglia
3. Both via hepatic plexus in the porta hepatis to accompany blood vessels and bile ducts

GALL BLADDER AND MAJOR BILE DUCTS
COMMON HEPATIC DUCT
1. Union of right and left hepatic ducts at porta hepatis
2. Joined by cystic duct 3 cm from parta
3. Lies on right of hepatic artery and in front of portal vein

GALLBLADDER
The gallbladder is a piriform sac lying in a fossa on the inferior surface of the liver and is attached to it by loose connective tissue. It is 7–10 cm in length and has a capacity of 30–50 ml.

Parts
1. Fundus
2. Body
3. Neck: Hartmans pouch may arise from neck

Cystic duct
1. 3–4 cm length
2. Joins hepatic duct to form common bile duct
3. Mucous membrane has crescenteric folds forming a spiral valve

COMMON BILE DUCT
The common bile duct is formed by the union of the common hepatic duct and the cystic duct. It is 7.5 cm long, 6 mm diameter. It joins the major pancreatic duct in the head of the pancreas to form the hepatopancreatic ampulla. This opens into the duodenum at the major duodenal papilla, 8–10 cm from the pylorus, on the posteromedial wall of the descending duodenum.

BLOOD SUPPLY
Gallbladder
Cystic artery dividing into superficial and deep branches

Common bile duct and hepatic duct
1. Upper part: cystic artery
2. Middle part
    a. right hepatic artery

    b. cystic artery
    c. posterior superior pancreaticoduodenal arteries
 3. Lower part: Posterior superior pancreaticoduodenal arteries

VENOUS DRAINAGE
Gallbladder
Direct into liver substance from upper surface. Two to three cystic veins direct to liver at porta hepatis.

Hepatic and bile ducts
 1. Upper part join with cystic veins and drain direct into liver
 2. Lower part direct into portal vein

LYMPHATIC DRAINAGE
 1. Upper surface of gallbladder: direct to liver
 2. Rest of gallbladder and upper part of bile ducts: Cystic node and porta hepatis nodes
 3. Lower part of bile ducts:
    1. Porta hepatitc nodes
    2. Lower hepatic nodes and upper pancreaticosplenic nodes

NERVE SUPPLY
 1. Autonomic via the coeliac plexus
 Autonomic plexuses lie in muscular and submucous layers of gallbladder and ducts

MICROSCOPIC STRUCTURE
Gallbladder
Layers
 1. Serous: Peritoneum and areolar tissue
 2. Fibromuscular: Smooth muscle which is longitudinal, circular and oblique
 3. Mucous:
    1. Absorptive columnar epithelium
    2. Few secretory mucous cells

Bile Ducts
Layers
 1. External: fibrous layer: fibroareolar tissue with a few smooth muscle fibres
 2. Internal:
    a. mucous layer: columnar epithelium
    b. tubulo-alveolar mucus-secreting glands

Sphincter of Oddi
This consists of a well-formed circular smooth muscle, which surrounds the lower end of the common bile duct, the terminal end of the pancreatic duct and the ampulla. It is continuous with the circular muscle of the duodenum.

PANCREAS
The pancreas is a soft lobulated organ, 15 cm in length. It lies transversely across the posterior abdominal wall behind the stomach and has both exocrine and endocrine function.

POSITION

Lies between duodenum and spleen, at the level of the transpyloric plane. The head occupies the C-shape of the duodenum in the right paravertebral gutter. It slopes slightly upwards across the posterior abdominal wall. The tail ends in the hilum of spleen.

STRUCTURE

Macroscopic
1. Head with uncinate process
2. Neck
3. Body
4. Tail
5. Main pancreatic duct receives tributaries in a herringbone manner. Joined by common bile duct in the head to form hepatopancreatic ampulla which opens into duodenum at major duodenal papilla
6. Accessory duct drains lower part of head and crosses main duct to open into duodenum proximally at the minor duodenal papilla

Microscopic

Parts
1. *Exocrine*
   a. acinar gland divided into lobules
   b. secretory cells: pyramidal shape arranged in flask-shaped groups which secrete inactive enzymes.
   c. ducts are lined by cuboidal and columnar cells.
   d. lobules divided up by loose connective tissue.
2. *Endocrine*
   1. Islets of Langerhans: clusters of cells embedded within exocrine part of pancreas. About 1 million cells per gland

2. Types of cell identified by staining:
   a. B: secrete Insulin
   b. A1: secrete Pancreatic gastrin
   c. A2: secrete Glucagon

The endothelial cells are fenestrated in the islets.

BLOOD SUPPLY

1. Superior and inferior pancreatico-duodenal arteries
2. Splenic artery by the arteria pancreatica magna and several short branches direct to the gland

VENOUS DRAINAGE

1. Superior pancreaticoduodenal vein to portal vein
2. Inferior pancreaticoduodenal vein to superior mesenteric vein
3. Multiple veins into splenic vein

LYMPHATIC DRAINAGE

Along arteries to pancreaticosplenic nodes, coeliac nodes and superior mesenteric preaortic nodes

NERVE SUPPLY

Autonomic via the coeliac and splenic plexuses
1. Parasympathetic: secretomotor ⎫ to exocrine pancreas
2. Sympathetic: vasomotor ⎭
3. Islets form part of neuro-endocrine complex
   Three types of nerve endings:
   a. cholinergic
   b. adrenergic
   c. non-identified type.

Genito-urinary system

URINARY SYSTEM: KIDNEYS

The two kidneys are retroperitoneal, lying high on the posterior abdominal wall, extending cranially to above the 12th rib.

POSITION

Lateral to the vertebral column between 12th thoracic and third lumbar vertebrae.

STRUCTURE

Macroscopic
1. Superior pole
2. Inferior pole
3. Hilum: on the right, it lies below the transpyloric plane; on the left, above it
4. Perirenal fat and fascia
5. Fibrous capsule
6. Cortex (outer part)
7. Medulla (inner part)

Microscopic
1. Nephron
   a. glomerulus
   b. renal tubule
      (i) proximal convoluted tubule
      (ii) loop of Henle
      (iii) distal convoluted tubule
2. Collecting tubules: collecting duct
3. Juxtaglomerular apparatus: juxtaglomerular cells in the wall of the afferent arteriole which lie in close contact with cells of the distal convoluted tubule

The glomeruli, proximal and distal tubules lie in the cortex, with the loops of Henle descending into the medulla.

COLLECTING SYSTEM

- Collecting duct
- Terminal duct of Bellini
- Renal papillae
- Minor calyx
- Major calyx
- Urinary pelvis

RENAL VASCULATURE

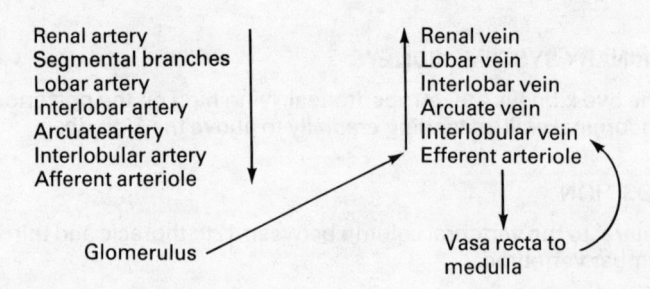

Renal artery → Segmental branches → Lobar artery → Interlobar artery → Arcuate artery → Interlobular artery → Afferent arteriole → Glomerulus → Efferent arteriole → Interlobular vein → Arcuate vein → Interlobar vein → Lobar vein → Renal vein

Vasa recta to medulla

Fig. 27 Renal vasculature.

NERVE SUPPLY

From the autonomic renal plexus. Mainly vasomotor

LYMPH DRAINAGE

Along the renal veins to the para-aortic lymph nodes

URETER

The ureter is a narrow muscular tube 25 cm long, which is divided into two equal portions: the abdominal part and the pelvic part. It is adherent to the overlying peritoneum.

POSITION

Abdominal part
1. Lies on psoas muscle
2. Crosses genitofemoral nerve
3. Crossed by gonadal vessels
4. Enters pelvis over bifurcation of common iliac artery, obturator nerve and sacro-iliac joint

Right ureter
Descends behind:
1. Second part of the duodenum
2. Right colic and ileocolic vessels
3. Root of the mesentery
4. Terminal part of ileum

Left ureter
Descends behind:
1. Left colic vessels
2. Root of sigmoid mesocolon

Pelvic part
1. Curves back in line with anterior border of greater sciatic notch
2. Descends over internal iliac vessels medial to their branches
3. Turns forward at level of ischial spines and then turns medially to enter lateral corners of the base of the bladder

In the male
Crosses ductus deferens laterally

In the female
Runs under the uterine artery, lateral to the cervix in the base of the broad ligament.

STRUCTURE
Macroscopic
1. Muscular tube
2. Narrows
   a. at pelvi-ureteric junction
   b. over pelvic brim
   c. on entry into the bladder

Microscopic
Transitional epithelium

Mucosa
1. Smooth and longitudinally folded
2. Continuous with renal papillae above and bladder below

Muscle coat
1. Upper two-thirds irregular
   a. inner longitudinal
   b. outer circular
2. Lower one-third has an additional outer longitudinal layer continuous with the bladder

Fibrous coat
1. Continuous above with the renal capsule
2. Merges with the extraperitoneal connective tissue and continues into the fibrous coat of the bladder

BLOOD SUPPLY AND LYMPHATIC DRAINAGE
Abdominal part
1. Renal, aortic and gonadal vessels
2. Para-aortic nodes

Pelvic part
1. Iliac, vesical and middle rectal vessels
2. Iliac nodes

NERVOUS SUPPLY
Autonomic from local plexuses

URINARY BLADDER
The urinary bladder is a reservoir for urine lying in the pelvis behind the pubic bones and anterior to the rectum. In the female, the vagina and uterus lie between the bladder and rectum, whereas in the male, the prostate and seminal vesicles lie in between.

STRUCTURE
Macroscopic
1. Base of fundus: alters shape with urinary volume
2. Trigone
   a. fixed to prostate in male
   b. fixed to anterior wall of vagina in female
3. Ureteric orifices (×2)
4. Interureteric fold: lies between ureteric orifices
5. Median umbilical ligament (urachus)
6. Medial umbilical ligaments (×2)
7. Lateral vesical ligaments (×2) (fascia lateral to bladder)

Microscopic
1. Serous layer (pelvic peritoneum)
2. Muscular layer: detrusor muscle (three layers); forms internal urethral sphincter
3. Mucosa: transitional epithelium

Genito-urinary system

BLOOD SUPPLY
1. Superior vesical artery
2. Inferior vesical artery

VENOUS DRAINAGE
Vesical plexus which drains to the internal iliac veins

LYMPH DRAINAGE
Along arteries to internal iliac lymph nodes

NERVE SUPPLY
Vesical plexus: contains sympathetic and parasympathetic fibres

Sympathetic fibres (11th thoracic to 2nd lumbar segments)
1. Stimulatory to internal sphincter
2. Inhibitory to detrusor muscle
3. Pain from bladder

Parasympathetic fibres
1. Stimulating to detrusor muscle
2. Inhibitory to internal sphincter
3. Pain from bladder
4. Awareness of bladder distension

URETHRA

MALE
This is approximately 20 cm long and extends from the bladder to the external opening (meatus) at the end of the penis. It is divided into three parts.

Parts

Prostatic urethra
1. 3 cm long and runs through prostate
2. Urethral crest (verumontanum) on posterior surface
3. Prostatic utricle lies in centre of urethral crest
4. Ejaculatory ducts open on side of utricle
5. Prostatic ducts open on each side of urethral crest

Membraneous urethra
1–2 cm long and surrounded by the sphincter urethrae

Spongiose urethra
1. 15 cm long contained within the corpus spongiosum
2. Dilated at each end
    a. the bulb (proximal)
    b. the navicular fossa (distal)
3. The bulbo-urethral glands open into it

Structure

Microscopic
1. Transitional epithelium from the bladder to ejaculatory ducts
2. Pseudostratified columnar epithelium to navicular fossa
3. Stratified squamous epithelium from navicular fossa to external urethral meatus

Vascular supply
This is derived from branches of the internal iliac artery and vein which supply the prostate and penis.

Nerve supply
Perineal branch of the pudendal nerve

Lymphatic drainage
1. Prostatic urethra ⎫ internal iliac
2. Membraneous urethra ⎭ nodes
3. Penile urethra
    a. deep inguinal nodes
    b. superficial inguinal nodes
    c. external iliac nodes

FEMALE

This is about 4 cm long and extends from the internal urethral orifice of the bladder to open anteriorly to the vagina. It lies within the anterior wall of the vagina and its opening is behind the glans clitoris.

Structure

Macroscopic
Similar to the male, with a posterior urethral crest and urethral glands. The para-urethral ducts open on each side of the external urethral orifice and are homologous to the prostate gland in the male.

Microscopic
Transitional epithelium near bladder which becomes stratified squamous epithelium distally.

Blood supply
From branches of the iliac artery and vein which supply the base of the bladder and anterior wall of vagina.

Nerve supply (sensation)
Perineal branch of the pudendal nerve

Lymphatic drainage
Internal iliac lymph nodes

MALE GENITAL SYSTEM:
TESTIS

The two testes lie within the scrotum, having descended through the inguinal canal from the posterior abdominal wall in the fetus. Their two main functions are spermatogenesis and hormone production.

STRUCTURE

Macroscopic
1. Tunica albuginae: fibrous capsule
2. Seminiferous tubules
3. Rete testis
4. Efferent duct
5. Epididymis
   a. head: lateral side of superior pole of testis on posterior surface
   b. body
   c. tail: inferior pole of testis

Microscopic
1. Seminiferous tubules
   a. spermatogonia
   b. supportive (sertoli) cells
   c. connective tissue
   d. interstitial Leydig cells (produce testosterone)
2. Efferent ductules: ciliated columnar epithelium
3. Epididymis: pseudostratified columnar epithelium (with microvilli)

BLOOD SUPPLY
1. Testicular artery
2. Testicular veins

LYMPH DRAINAGE

Along testicular artery to para-aortic lymph nodes

NERVE SUPPLY

1. Sympathetic supply from renal and aortic plexus (derived from 11th and 12th thoracic segments of the spinal cord) is vasomotor and sensory
2. Parasympathetic supply from the inferior hypogastric plexus is vasodilator

DUCTUS DEFERENS (VAS DEFERENS)

The vas deferens runs from the tail of the epididymis up the medial side of the testis. It traverses the inguinal canal in the spermatic cord to enter the pelvis at the deep inguinal ring, from where it crosses the external iliac vessels, obturator vessels and ureter before reaching the seminal vesicles. They are dilated to form ampullae before entering the seminal vesicles.

STRUCTURE

Microscopic
1. Non-ciliated columnar epithelium
2. Thick muscular wall

ARTERIAL SUPPLY

1. Artery to ductus deferens (branch of inferior vesical artery)
2. Anastomoses with artery to epididymis which is a branch of the testicular artery

VENOUS DRAINAGE

To inferior vesical veins

LYMPHATIC DRAINAGE

External iliac lymph nodes

NERVE SUPPLY

Autonomic fibres from pelvic plexuses

SEMINAL VESICLES

These are two saccules placed between the posterior surface of the bladder and the rectum, which join on the superior surface of the prostate to form the ejaculatory ducts.

Genito-urinary system

STRUCTURE

Microscopic
Columnar epithelium with diverticuli containing goblet cells

VASCULAR SUPPLY
From branches of the internal vesical and middle rectal vessels

LYMPHATIC DRAINAGE
Internal and external iliac lymph nodes

NERVE SUPPLY
Autonomic fibres from the pelvic plexuses

SPERMATIC CORD
The spermatic cord consists of structures taken through the inguinal ligament with the testis as it descends into the scrotum.

STRUCTURES
1. Ductus deferens
2. Testicular artery
3. Cremasteric artery
4. Deferential artery (to ductus deferens)
5. Testicular veins
6. Lymph vessels
7. Genital branch of genitofemoral nerve
8. Testicular plexus of autonomic fibres

Coverings
1. External spermatic fascia (derived from external oblique)
2. Cremasteric fascia (derived from internal oblique)
3. Internal spermatic fascia (derived from transversalis fascia)

SCROTUM
The scrotum is a sac which contains the testes, which are separated from each other by a sagittal septum.

STRUCTURE
1. Skin
2. Dartos muscle (supplied by sympathetic fibres in the genitofemoral nerve)

3. External spermatic fascia
4. Cremasteric fascia
5. Internal spermatic fascia
6. Tunica vaginalis

ARTERIAL SUPPLY
1. External pudendal branches of femoral artery
2. Scrotal branches of internal pudendal artery
3. Cremasteric branch of inferior epigastric artery

VENOUS DRAINAGE
Follows arteries

LYMPHATIC DRAINAGE
Inguinal lymph nodes

NERVE SUPPLY
1. Ilioinguinal nerve
2. Genital branch of genitofemoral nerve
3. Posterior scrotal branches of perineal nerve
4. Perineal branch of posterior cutaneous nerve of thigh.

PENIS
The penis is attached by its root to the margins of the pubic arch and the intervening perineal membrane.

STRUCTURE
Root
1. Bulb of penis and bulbospongiosum (becomes corpus spongiosum)
2. Crura of penis and ischiocavernosi (become corpora cavernosa)

Body
1. Corpus spongiosum supported by the ischiocavernosi muscles and the suspensory ligament
2. Corpora cavernosa
3. Tunica albuginea: superficial and deep fibrous layers which surround the erectile tissue of the penis. It also forms the septum which divides the two corpora

Glans

Urethra
Within the corpus spongiosum

ARTERIAL SUPPLY

1. Dorsal arteries of penis
2. Deep arteries of penis

VENOUS SUPPLY

Dorsal veins of penis

LYMPHATIC DRAINAGE

1. Superficial inguinal nodes
2. Deep inguinal nodes } glans penis
3. External iliac nodes

NERVE SUPPLY

1. Dorsal nerve of penis (branch of pudendal nerve)
2. Autonomic fibres from pelvic plexuses

PROSTATE
The prostate is a small, firm gland which surrounds the commencement of the urethra in the male.

STRUCTURE

Macroscopic
1. Apex (inferior)
2. Median lobe
3. Right and left lobes
4. Contains urethra and ejaculatory ducts

Microscopic
1. Fibrous sheath
2. Muscular stroma
3. Glandular substance: follicles and excretory ducts

ARTERIAL SUPPLY

Branches of
1. Internal pudendal artery
2. Inferior vesical artery
3. Middle rectal artery

VENOUS DRAINAGE

Prostatic venous plexus around sides of gland which drain to the internal iliac veins.

LYMPHATIC DRAINAGE

Internal iliac lymph nodes

NERVE SUPPLY

Autonomic fibres from pelvic plexuses

ERECTION AND EJACULATION

ERECTION

This is brought about by increased arterial flow into the erectile tissue of the corpora cavernosa of the penis.

EJACULATION

This consists of several parts:
1. Contraction of seminal vesicles
2. Seminal ejaculation
3. Contraction of internal urethral sphincter
4. Inhibition of bladder musculature

The autonomic nervous mechanisms involved are complex. It is thought that parasympathetic fibres initiate erection and contraction of the seminal vesicles, while sympathetic fibres stimulate seminal ejaculation with inhibition of bladder musculature and contraction of the internal sphincter to prevent reflux of the ejaculate into the bladder.

FEMALE GENITAL SYSTEM

OVARY

The ovaries are homologous to the testes in the male. They lie close to the lateral walls of the pelvis overlying the obturator vessels, in the ovarian fossa. They are connected to the fallopian tubes on each side by the ovarian fimbria and to the uterus posteriorly by the ovarian ligaments.

STRUCTURE

Microscopic
1. Outer germinal epithelium
2. Tunica albuginea
3. Ovarian follicles
4. Interstitial stroma

VASCULAR SUPPLY
1. Ovarian artery
2. Ovarian vein

LYMPHATIC DRAINAGE
Para-aortic lymph nodes

NERVE SUPPLY
Autonomic fibres from aortic and pelvic plexuses

FALLOPIAN TUBE
The fallopian (uterine) tubes transmit ova from the ovaries to the uterus. They are situated in the upper parts of the broad ligaments.

STRUCTURE
Macroscopic
1. Infundibulum: dilated ovarian end
2. Fimbria: processes extending from infundibulum
3. Ampulla: middle part of tube
4. Isthmus: medial one-third of tube
5. Uterine part: this is intramural

Macroscopic
1. External serosal layer
2. Intermediate muscle layer
3. Mucous membrane: ciliated columnar epithelium arranged in many folds

VASCULAR SUPPLY
1. Ovarian artery (lateral one-third)
2. Uterine artery (medial two-thirds)
3. Ovarian vein
4. Uterine vein

LYMPHATIC DRAINAGE
1. Para-aortic lymph nodes
2. External iliac lymph nodes (uterine part of tube)

NERVE SUPPLY
Autonomic fibres from aortic and pelvic plexuses

UTERUS

The uterus is a hollow muscular organ which lies in the pelvis between the bladder and rectum. It can be anteverted (lying with the fundus facing anterior) or retroverted (the fundus facing posterior).

STRUCTURE

Macroscopic
1. Fundus
2. Body
3. Cervix uteri
4. Cavity

Microscopic
1. External serous layer (peritoneum)
2. Middle muscular layer (non-striated fibres)
3. Columnar epithelium

The mucous membrane of the cervix uteri contains numerous glands and changes from ciliated columnar in the upper two-thirds to stratified squamous in the lower one-third.

VASCULAR SUPPLY

1. Uterine arteries
2. Uterine veins

LYMPHATIC DRAINAGE

1. External and internal iliac lymph nodes
2. Para-aortic lymph nodes
3. Superficial inguinal lymph nodes

NERVE SUPPLY

Autonomic fibres from aortic and pelvic plexuses

UTERINE LIGAMENTS

BROAD LIGAMENT

1. Infundibulopelvic fold: ovary to lateral wall of pelvis
2. Mesosalpynx: between fallopian tube and ovarian ligament
3. Mesovarium: attaches ovary to posterior layer of broad ligament
4. Contents:
    a. fallopian tube
    b. ovarian artery
    c. uterine artery
    d. ovarian ligament (ovary to uterus)

ROUND LIGAMENT
Continuation of ovarian ligament through deep inguinal ring to inguinal canal and inserts into labia majora (remnant of Gubernaculum)

LATERAL LIGAMENT (OF MACKENDRODT)
Cervix to lateral walls of pelvis

UTEROSACRAL LIGAMENTS
Cervix uteri to sacrum on each side of rectum

ANTERIOR LIGAMENT
Formed by peritoneum of uterovesical fold

POSTERIOR LIGAMENT
Formed by peritoneum of rectovaginal fold

VAGINA
The vagina is a fibromuscular tube which extends from the labia minora to the cervix. It is situated between the bladder and urethra (anteriorly) and the rectum (posteriorly). Deep on each side lie the fibres of pubovaginalis and its superficial part is surrounded by bulbospongiosus.

The vagina is separated from the bladder by the uterovesical pouch, and from the rectum by the recto-uterine pouch (of Douglas). The perineal body separates the lower part of the vagina from the anal canal.

STRUCTURE
Microscopic
1. Stratified squamous epithelium
2. Non-striated muscle fibres

ARTERIAL SUPPLY
1. Vaginal artery
2. Uterine artery
3. Internal pudendal artery
4. Middle rectal artery

VENOUS DRAINAGE
1. Venous plexus around vagina to internal iliac veins

LYMPHATIC DRAINAGE
External and internal iliac lymph nodes

EXTERNAL GENITAL ORGANS

PARTS

Mons pubis
Formed by subcutaneous adipose tissue in front of the symphysis pubis

Labia majora
1. Homologous to scrotum in the male
2. Outer folds surrounding vaginal orifice
3. Round ligament ends

Labia minora
1. Cutaneous folds which lie within the labia majora
2. At its upper end it forms prepuce of clitoris (above clitoris) and frenulum of clitoris (below clitoris)

Vestibule
1. Cleft between labia minora
2. Contains vaginal and urethral orifices
3. Vestibular (Bartholin's) glands open on each side

Clitoris
1. Erectile structure (homologous to penis)
2. Enclosed by anterior folds of labia minora
3. Body (corpora cavernosa) supported by ischiocavernosa muscles
4. Glans

Vaginal orifice (introitus)
Between labia minora

Hymen
Thin fold of mucous membrane around orifice of vagina

Bulbs of vestibule
1. Formed by erectile tissue on each side of the vaginal orifice (homologous to bulb of penis in male)
2. Covered superficially by bulbospongiosus muscles

Genito-urinary system

VASCULAR SUPPLY
Similar to those supplying the homologous structures in the male:
1. Internal pudendal artery
2. External pudendal arteries (two on each side)
3. Venous drainage to external and internal iliac veins

LYMPHATIC DRAINAGE
1. Superficial inguinal lymph nodes
2. Clitoris drains to lymph node of Cloquet (deep inguinal lymph nodes)

NERVE SUPPLY
1. Autonomic from pelvic plexuses
2. Sensory
   a. Ilio-inguinal nerve
   b. Dorsal nerve of clitoris
   c. Perineal branch (of posterior femoral cutaneous nerve of thigh)
   d. Genital branch (of genitofemoral nerve)
   e. Perineal branch (of pudendal nerve)

EMBRYOLOGICAL DERIVATIONS OF THE GENITO-URINARY TRACT

KIDNEY
Metanephros

URETER
Grows out from mesonephric duct

VAS DEFERENS
Mesonephric duct (Wolfian duct)

EPOOPHORON, PAROOPHORON, GARTNER'S DUCT
Vestigial structures from the mesonephric duct in the female

VAS EFFERENS (AND APPENDICES)
Mesonephric tubules

VAGINA
Mullerian duct

CERVIX
UTERUS } MULLERIAN DUCT
FALLOPIAN TUBES
PROSTATIC UTRICLE, APPENDIX OF TESTIS
Vestigial remnants of Mullerian duct in the male

BLADDER
1. Anterior part of cloaca (urogenital sinus)
2. Mesonephric duct
3. Urogenital sinus
4. Ectoderm

Peritoneum

The peritoneum is a serous membrane consisting of a closed sac. Part of this lines the abdominal wall (parietal) whilst the remainder is reflected over the contained viscera (visceral). In the female this sac is deficient where the fallopian tube opens into the peritoneal cavity. Structures in the abdomen may be intra- or extraperitoneal, with the area posterior to the peritoneum of the posterior abdominal wall called the retroperitoneum.

BOUNDARIES OF PERITONEAL CAVITY

Although all structures, both intra- and extraperitoneal, will be described under their various systems, it is worth mentioning the boundaries of the peritoneal cavity:

Superior
Diaphragm

Posterior
Posterior abdominal wall:
1. Quadratus lumborum
2. Psoas
3. Vertebral column

Antero-lateral
Muscles of anterior abdominal wall

Anterior
Rectus muscle and posterior rectus sheath (down to the semicircular fold of Douglas)

Inferior
Pelvic diaphragm (levator ani)

NERVE AND BLOOD SUPPLY

Parietal: somatic nerves and vessels

Visceral: Vessels and autonomic nerves supplying the associated viscera.

PERITONEAL FOLDS

GREATER OMENTUM

Develops from dorsal mesogastrium

Gastrocolic omentum
Greater curve of stomach to the transverse colon

Gastrophrenic ligament
Fundus of stomach to the diaphragm (above the spleen)

Gastrosplenic ligament
Greater curve of stomach to the spleen

Lienorenal ligament
Spleen to the left kidney
The greater omentum continues over the transverse colon to cover the viscera.

LESSER OMENTUM

Develops from ventral mesogastrium

Hepatogastric ligament
Lesser curve of stomach to liver

Hepatoduodenal ligament
Liver to 1st part of duodenum

EPIPLOIC FORAMEN

Connects the greater and lesser sacs (3 cm long).

Anterior
Right margin of lesser omentum with:
 1. Common bile duct (right)
 2. Hepatic artery (left)
 3. Portal vein (posterior)

Superior
Caudate process of liver (with posterior layer of right margin of lesser omentum).

Peritoneum

Posterior
Inferior vena cava (covered by parietal peritoneum which is still a continuation of the posterior layer of the right margin of the lesser omentum).

Floor
The continuation of the same layer of peritoneum.

HEPATIC FOLDS

Falciform ligament
Containing the ligamentum teres which is the obliterated left umbilical vein.

Coronary ligament

Left and Right triangular ligaments

Hepatorenal pouch (of Rutherford Morrison)

Right margin of the lesser omentum

PELVIC FOLDS

1. Rectovesical pouch (and fascia of Denonvilliers)
2. Recto-uterine pouch of Douglas
3. Broad ligament contains
    a. round ligament
    b. ovarian ligament
    c. ovary (on its mesovarium)
    d. fallopian tube and vessels
    e. mesometrium (contains uterine artery inferiorly)
4. Infundibulopelvic fold
   Ovary to side wall of pelvis (contains ovarian artery)
5. Vesico-uterine pouch

MESENTERIES

Reflections of peritoneum from the posterior abdominal wall, which invest the bowel, and through which the blood supply, venous and lymphatic drainage of the bowel run.
The mesenteries of the stomach are the greater and lesser omenti.

Small bowel mesentery
Root
1. 15 cm long
2. From duodenojejunal flexure (level of L2) to upper part of right sacroiliac joint

Paraduodenal recesses
1. Superior duodenal recess
2. Inferior duodenal recess
3. Paraduodenal recess
4. Retroduodenal recess

Ileocaecal folds
1. Mesoappendix
2. Avascular fold of Treves (ileocaecal fold)
3. Vascular fold of caecum
4. Retrocaecal recess

Mesocolon
Mesentery of the transverse colon (attaches to left diaphragm as phrenicocolic ligament).

Sigmoid mesocolon

Mesorectum

DEVELOPMENTAL FOLDS
1. Median umbilical fold (urachus)
2. Right and Left medial umbilical folds, (from the umbilical arteries, the proximal part remains as the superior vesical artery)
3. Lateral umbilical folds (inferior epigastric artery)
4. Falciform ligament (see p. 125).

Myology

Muscle cells develop mainly from mesenchyme, into three different types:
1. Skeletal ⎫ Striated
2. Cardiac ⎭
3. Smooth   Non striated.

Cardiac muscle is described in Chapter 1. Skeletal muscle only will be described here.

SKELETAL MUSCLE
STRUCTURE

Muscle
Fibres made up of multinucleate cells whose length vary considerably. Arranged in fasiculi (bundles). The entire muscle is made up of numerous fasiculi. Each muscle is surrounded with a connective tissue layer the epimysium.

Tendons
Integral parts of a muscle of unvarying length. Made of longitudinally arranged collagen bundles often interwoven. Attach the muscle to its bony insertion.

Aponeuroses
Flat sheets of densely arranged collagen fibres. May spread from the edge of a tendon to provide an extension of insertion. May form the major part of the insertion. May provide extra surface from which muscle fibres may arise.

Fascia
Condensations of connective tissue between structures and muscular planes of the body.

Superficial fascia
Loose areolar tissue beneath the dermis. Allows the skin freedom of movement and acts as a thermal insulator.

Deep fascia
Dense arrangement of collagen fibres which enclose muscle and fuse to underlying bone. Forms the intermuscular septa and retinaculi.

Bursae
Flattened sacs of synovium, which allow free movement of tissues on either side.

Synovial sheaths
Cylindrical double-layered sheaths of synovium surrounding tendons. Visceral layer attached to the tendon and a parietal layer attached to the surrounding tissues. With bursae these occur in areas where structures in close proximity move relative to each other.

BLOOD AND NERVE SUPPLY
The neurovascular bundle enters at the neurovascular hiatus which is usually one-third from its origin.

TYPES OF MUSCLE

Quadrilateral	Thyrohyoid
Strap	Sternohyoid, sartorius, rectus abdominis
Fusiform	Biceps brachii
Digastric	Digastric, omohyoid
Tricipital	Triceps
Triangular	Temporalis, adductor longus
Circumpennate	Tibialis anterior
Spiral	Latissimus dorsi
Cruciate	Adductor magnus, masseter
Unipennate	Flexor pollicis longus
Bipennate	Rectus femoris, dorsal interossei
Multipennate	Deltoid

ACTION OF MUCSLE
Muscle may be active and develop tension when at a fixed length, shortening or lengthening. May act as:
1. Prime movers
2. Antagonists
3. Synergists

Antagonists oppose prime movers. Synergists assist the prime mover to ensure a smooth action. Opposing groups of muscles may fix one joint to allow movement at another.

Joint movement is described in its component parts and the actions of muscles are described in a similar way.

Myology

PAGES 130–171

Tables of individual muscles are described under the following headings:

Muscles of the head, mouth, palate and pharynx

Muscles of the neck
Muscles of the trunk
Muscles of the thorax
Muscles of the abdomen
Muscles of the pelvis
Muscles of the perineum
Muscles of the upper limb
Muscles of the lower limb

ABBREVIATIONS

Transverse process, TP.
Vertebrae and nerve roots referred to as C, T, L, S, according to cervical, thoracic, lumbar and sacral positions. Numbers refer to level.

MUSCLES OF THE HEAD, MOUTH, PALATE AND PHARYNX

Muscles of the face (excluding small intrinsic muscles)

Muscle	Origin	Insertion	Nerve supply	Action
Occipitofrontalis	Two occipital bellies Each arises from lateral two-thirds superior nuchal line and mastoid part of temporal bone Connected by epicranial aponeurosis to frontal bellies	Two frontal bellies No bony insertion Blend with proceros, orbicularis oculi and corrugator supercilli	Occipital belly by posterior auricular branch, and frontal belly by temporal branch of the facial nerve	Draws scalp backward and wrinkles forehead; raises eyebrows
Orbicularis oculi (three parts)	*Orbital:* nasal part of frontal bone; frontal process of maxilla; medial palpebral ligament	Complete ellipse round eye	Temporal and zygomatic branches of facial nerve	Sphincter of the eye. *Orbital:* voluntary control *Palpebral:* involuntary control *Lacrimal:* dilates lacrimal sac
	Palpebral: medial palpebral ligament	Elliptical path round eye and forms lateral palpebral raphe		
	Lacrimal: lacrimal bone adjacent to lacrimal sac	Lateral palpebral raphe		

Buccinator	Outer surface of alveolar processes of maxilla and mandible opposite the three molar teeth; pterygomandibular ligament	Intersects with fibres of orbicularis oris	Buccal branches of facial nerve	Keeps cheeks against teeth
Orbicularis oris	Fibres from other facial muscles coming in towards the angles of mouth. Fibres attaching lips to maxilla above and the mandible below. Fibres running obliquely across lips	Inserted into lips	Buccal and mandibular branches of facial nerve	Deep part compresses lips against teeth Superficial part brings lips together

Muscles of mastication

Muscle	Origin	Insertion	Nerve supply	Action
Masseter (three parts)	*Superficial*: zygomatic process of maxilla. Anterior two-thirds lower border of zygomatic arch	Angle and lower half of lateral surface of ramus of mandible	Branch of anterior trunk of mandibular nerve	Elevates mandible against maxilla i.e. occludes teeth
	Middle: deep surface anterior two-thirds and lower border of posterior one-third of the zygomatic arch	Coronoid process and upper half ramus of mandible		
	Deep: deep surface of zygomatic arch	Middle of ramus of mandible		
Temporalis	Temporal fossa and deep surface of temporal fascia	Coronoid process and anterior border of ramus of mandible to 1st molar tooth	Deep temporal branch of anterior trunk of mandibular nerve	Closes the mouth. Retraction of mandible
Lateral pterygoid (two heads)	*Upper*: infratemporal surface of greater wing of sphenoid. *Lower*: lateral surface of lateral pterygoid plate	Front of neck of mandible. Articular disc of temporomandibular joint	Branch of anterior trunk of mandibular nerve	Opens mouth. Protrudes mandible with medial pterygoid
Medial pterygoid	Medial surface of lateral pterygoid plate. Pyramidal process of the palatine bone	Lower and back part medial surface of ramus and angle of mandible	Branch of the mandibular nerve	Protrusion with lateral pterygoid. Chewing movement when acting with lateral pterygoid unilaterally

Muscles of the tongue

Genioglossus	Upper genial tubercle on inner surface of mandibular symphysis	Anterior surface of body of hyoid. Ventral surface of tongue from root to apex	Hypoglossal nerve	Pulls tongue forward and protrudes it out of mouth. Makes tongue concave side to side
Hypoglossus	Greater horn and lateral part of body, of hyoid bone	Side of tongue	Hypoglossal nerve	Depress tongue
Chondroglossus	Lesser horn and adjacent part of body, of hyoid bone	Side of tongue	Hypoglossal nerve	Depress tongue
Styloglossus	Apex of styloid process and stylomandibular ligament	Dorsal surface of tongue	Hypoglossal nerve	Draws tongue upwards and backwards

Muscles of pharynx

Stylopharyngeus	Base of styloid process	Posterior border of thyroid cartilage with palatopharyngeus	Glossopharyngeal nerve	Elevator of pharynx in swallowing and speech
Salpingopharyngeus	Cartilaginous inferior part of internal auditory tube	Blends with palatopharyngeus	Pharyngeal plexus	Raises pharynx in swallowing

Muscles of the palate

Muscle	Origin	Insertion	Nerve supply	Action
Levator veli palatini	Inferior surface of petrous temporal bone; fascia arising from vaginal process of tympanic part of temporal bone	Upper surface of palatine aponeurosis blends with its opposite number in midline		Elevates the soft palate
Tensor veli palatini (TVP)	Inferior surface of cartilaginous part of auditory tube Scaphoid fossa of pterygoid process Cartilage of auditory tube Spine of sphenoid bone	Small tendon turns round the pterygoid hamulus. Palatine aponeurosis and horizontal plate of pterygoid bone	Nucleus ambiguus via accessory nerve and thence via vagus to pharyngeal plexus Except TVP: mandibular nerve via nerve to medial pterygoid	Unilateral: pulls palate to one side Together: flattens and tightens the palate
Musculus uvulae: bilateral structure	Posterior nasal spine of palatine bones Palatine aponeurosis	Mucous membrane of uvula		Pulls up uvula
Palatoglossus	Oral surface of palatine aponeurosis Continuous with its opposite number in the midline	Side of tongue: dorsum and deeply		Together: closes off mouth from oropharynx

Palatopharyngeus (two fasciculi)	*Anterior:* posterior border of hard palate and palatine aponeurosis	Posterior border of thyroid cartilage. Few fibres into pharyngeal wall	Together approximate palatopharyngeal arches. Shorten pharynx during swallowing
	Posterior: pharyngeal surface of palatine aponeurosis		

Suprahyoid and infrahyoid muscles

Muscle	Origin	Insertion	Nerve supply	Action
Digastric	Two bellies united by tendon attached to the hyoid bone by a fibrous loop: *Posterior belly*: arises from mastoid notch of temporal bone *Anterior belly*: arises from digastric fossa of mandible		*Posterior belly*: facial nerve *Anterior belly*: mylohyoid branch of inferior alveolar nerve	Act together to elevate hyoid bone and depress the mandible
Stylohyoid	Base of styloid process	Body of hyoid bone	Facial nerve	Elevates and draws back the hyoid
Mylohyoid	Mylohyoid line of mandible	Body of hyoid Midline raphe from hyoid to symphysis menti	Mylohyoid branch of inferior alveolar nerve	Elevates the floor of the mouth
Geniohyoid	Inferior mental spine of symphysis menti	Anterior surface of body of hyoid	1st cervical nerve via the hypoglossal nerve	Elevates and draws forward the hyoid
Sternohyoid	Posterior surface of medial end of clavicle Posterior aspect of sternoclavicular ligament and manubrium	Lower border of body of hyoid	Ansa cervicalis	Depresses hyoid bone
Sternothyroid	Posterior surface of manubrium 1st costal cartilage	Oblique line on lamina of thyroid cartilage	Ansa cervicalis	Draws larynx downward
Thyrohyoid	Oblique line on lamina of thyroid cartilage	Lower border of greater cornu of hyoid bone	1st cervical nerve via the hypoglossal nerve	Depresses hyoid, raises larynx

Myology 137

Muscle	Origin	Insertion	Nerve supply	Action
Omohyoid	Two bellies united by a central tendon lying adjacent to the internal jugular vein opposite cricoid cartilage held by a band of fibrous tissue to clavicle and 1st rib: *Inferior belly*: upper border of scapula adjacent to suprascapular notch *Superior belly*: lower border of body of hyoid bone		*Inferior belly*: ansa cervicalis *Superior belly*: ramus superior of ansa cervicalis	Depresses hyoid

Anterior and lateral vertebral muscles

Muscle	Origin	Insertion	Nerve supply	Action
Longus colli (three parts)	*Inferior oblique:* anterior aspect vertebral bodies T1–T3 *Superior oblique:* anterior tubercles of TPs C3–C5 *Vertical:* anterior aspect vertebral bodies C5–T3	Anterior tubercles of TPs C5, C6 Tubercle on anterior arch of atlas Anterior aspect vertebral bodies C2–C4	ventral rami of C2–C6 nerves	Flexion, lateral flexion and rotation of cervical spine
Longus capitis	Anterior tubercles TPs C3–C6	Inferior surface basilar part of occipital bone	Ventral rami C1–C3	Flex the head
Rectus capitis anterior	Anterior surface of lateral mass of atlas	Inferior surface basilar part of occipital bone	Ventral rami C1–C2	Flex the head
Rectus capitis lateralis	TP of atlas	Inferior surface of jugular process of occipital bone	Ventral rami C1–C2	Bend head to same side
Scalenus Anterior	Anterior tubercles of TPs C3–C6	Scalene tubercle of 1st rib	Ventral rami C4–C6	Flexion, lateral flexion and rotation to opposite side of cervical spine — all act as accessory muscles of respiration
Scalenus Medius	TP of axis Posterior tubercles of TPs C3–C7	Upper surface of 1st rib	Ventral rami C3–C8	Lateral flexion of cervical spine — all act as accessory muscles of respiration
Scalenus Posterior	Posterior tubercles of TPs C4–C6	Outer surface of 2nd rib	Ventral rami C6–C8	Lateral flexion of cervical spine — all act as accessory muscles of respiration

MUSCLES OF THE NECK

Superficial group

Muscle	Origin	Insertion	Nerve supply	Action
Platysma	Fascia covering deltoid and pectoralis major	Lower border of body of mandible Skin and subcutaneous tissue on lower part of face	Cervical branch of facial nerve	Wrinkles skin of neck Draws lower lip down
Sternocleidomastoid (two heads)	*Sternal:* upper part anterior surface of manubrium *Clavicular:* upper surface of medial one-third of clavicle Two heads unite into single tendon	Lateral surface of mastoid process Lateral half of superior nuchal line	*Motor:* accessory nerve *Sensory:* branches of C2, C3 ventral rami, from cervical plexus	Tilts head to same side and rotates face to opposite side Together flex cervical cervical spine Accessory muscle of respiration

MUSCLES OF TRUNK

Muscles of the back

Muscle	Origin	Insertion	Nerve supply	Action
Splenius capitis	Lower half ligamentum nuchae Spines of C7–T4	Mastoid process of temporal bone Occipital bone below lateral one-third superior nuchal line	Dorsal rami of middle cervical nerves	Draw head back when all four act together Rotate head to same side when two splenii on one side act together
Splenius cervicis	Spines of T3–T6	Posterior tubercles of TPs C3–C4	Dorsal rami of lower cervical nerves	
Sacrospinalis	Common origin from a broad tendon arising from median crest of sacrum, spines and supraspinous ligaments of T11–L5 Medial part of iliac crest Lateral crest of sacrum and sacrotuberous ligament	Divides into three vertical columns in the lumbar region Lateral, intermediate and medial		

Lateral column: iliocostalis (three parts)	*Iliocostalis lumborum:* Common origin	Inferior border of angles of lower seven ribs	dorsal rami cervical, thoracic and lumbar nerves
	Iliocostalis thoracis: Upper borders of angles of lower six ribs	Upper borders of upper six ribs	Extension and lateral flexion of vertebral column
	Iliocostalis cervicis: angles of third to sixth ribs	Posterior tubercles TPs of C4–C6	
Intermediate column: longissimus (three parts)	*Longissimus thoracis* Continuation of sacrospinalis. Posterior surfaces of TPs and accessory processes of lumbar vertebrae	Tips of TPs of thoracic vertebrae. Lower nine ribs between tubercles and angles	Dorsal rami of cervical thoracic and lumbar nerves
	Longissimus cervicis TPs of upper four or five thoracic vertebrae	Posterior tubercles TPs of C2–C6	Extension and lateral flexion of spine
	Longissimus capitis TPs of upper four to five thoracic vertebrae Articular processes of lower three to four cervical vertebrae	Mastoid process	Extends head

Aids to anatomy

Muscle	Origin	Insertion	Nerve supply	Action
Medial column: spinalis (two parts)	*Spinalis thoracis*: Continuation of sacrospinalis, and spines of T11–L2	Spines of upper four to eight thoracic vertebrae	Dorsal rami of cervical and thoracic nerves	Extend vertebral column
	Spinalis cervicis: Lower part of ligamentum nuchae Spine of C7	Spine of axis		
Transverso spinalis: group of muscles originating on transverse processes and inserting on spines of vertebrae (three parts)				
	Semispinalis thoracis: TPs of T6–T10	Spines of C6–T4	Dorsal rami of cervical and thoracic nerves	Extends and rotates vertebral column
	Semispinalis cervicis: TPs of T1–T6	Spines of C2–C5		
	Semispinalis capitis: Tips of TPs C7–T7 Articular processes C4–C6	Medial part of area between inferior and superior nuchal lines		Extends and rotates head
Multifidus	Back of sacrum from 4th foramen upwards Mamillary processes of lumbar vertebrae Transverse processes of thoracic vertebrae Articular processes of lower four cervical vertebrae	Spinous process of vertebra three levels above origin Highest level C2	Dorsal rami of spinal nerves	Postural muscles Maintain posture and structural integrity of vertebral column and allow long muscles to function
Rotatores (only in thoracic region 11 in number on each side)	Upper posterior part of TP	Lower border lamina next vertebrae above	Dorsal rami of thoracic nerves	

Interspinales	Run between spines of contiguous vertebrae in cervical thoracic and lumbar region		Dorsal rami of spinal nerves
Intertransversarii	Run between transverse processes of adjacent vertebrae. Cervical to lumbar region		Dorsal and ventral rami of spinal nerves

Suboccipital muscles

Rectus capitis posterior major	Spine of axis	Lateral part of inferior nuchal line	Dorsal ramus of 1st spinal nerve
			Extends head
			Turns head same way
Rectus capitis posterior minor	Tubercle on posterior arch of atlas	Medial part of inferior nuchal line	Extends head
Obliquus capitis superior	Upper surface TP of atlas	Area between inferior and superior nuchal lines	Extends head
			Turns head same side
Obliquus capitis inferior	Lateral surface of spine of axis	TP of the atlas	Turns head same side

Myology 143

MUSCLES OF THE THORAX

Muscle	Origin	Insertion	Nerve supply	Action
External intercostals (11 on each side)	Lower border of rib Each muscle extends from tubercle of rib to become continuous with anterior/external intercostal membrane anteriorly adjacent to costal cartilages	Upper border of rib below Fibres pass obliquely down and laterally at the back; down and forwards at the front	Corresponding intercostal nerve	Respiration by elevation and eversion of the ribs, to increase transverse and A-P diameter of the thorax
Internal intercostals (11 on each side)	Lower border of rib Each muscle extends from sternum anteriorly, to angles of rib posteriorly to become continuous with internal intercostal membrane	Upper border of rib below Fibres pass obliquely down at right angles to external intercostals	As above	
Subcostales	Inner surface of rib at its angle. Fibres pass in same direction as internal intercostals	Inner surface of rib two to three levels lower	As above	Respiration: depressing ribs
Intercostales intimi	Inner surface of rib Covers middle half of intercostal space	Inner surface of rib below	As above	With internal intercostals
Transversus thoracis (Sternocostalis)	Lower one-third posterior surface of sternum Posterior surface of xiphoid Post surface of lower two to three true costal cartilages	Lower borders and inner surface of costal cartilages 2nd–6th ribs	As above	Draws down costal cartilages

Muscle	Origin	Insertion	Nerve supply	Action
Levatores costarum (12 on each side)	Tips of TPs C7–T11	Between tubercle and angle of upper outer surface of rib below vertebral level of origin	Dorsal rami segmentally	Respiration: elevate the ribs
Serratus posterior superior	Lower part ligamentum nuchae; spines and supraspinous ligaments of C7–T2(3)	Upper outer surface of 2–5th ribs, lateral to its angle	2nd–5th intercostal nerves	Elevates ribs
Serratus posterior inferior	Spines and supraspinous ligaments of T11–L2	Lower outer surface of lowest four ribs lateral to angles	Ventral rami 9–12 thoracic nerves	Draws lower ribs down Fixes diaphragm
Diaphragm (three parts)	*Sternal*: two slips from xiphoid process *Costal*: internal surfaces of lower six ribs and costal cartilages *Lumbar*: consists of a. lateral lumbocostal arch (lateral arcuate ligament) from 12th rib and TP of L1 b. medial lumbocostal arch (medial arcuate ligament) from bodies L1, L2 c. right crus from sides and discs of vertebral bodies L1–L3 d. left crus from sides and discs of vertebral bodies L1, L2	Central tendon Trilobar shape: middle leaf with apex towards xiphoid; right and left leaves run backward and laterally	*Motor*: phrenic nerves C3–C5 *Sensory*: segmental from lowest intercostal nerves	During inspiration the central tendon is drawn downwards. Once abdominal movement ceases the central tendon becomes fixed. The peripheral fibres then act to elevate the ribs and push out the sternum

MUSCLES OF THE ABDOMEN

Muscles	Origin	Insertion	Nerve supply	Action
Obliquus externus abdominis (external oblique)	Eight fleshy digitations from outer, anterior surface of lowest eight ribs at their anterior angles, interdigitate with origin of latissimus dorsi and serratus anterior. Muscle becomes aponeurotic on a line from 9th costal cartilage vertically to level of umbilicus and then laterally to anterior superior iliac spine (ASIS)	Inferior and laterally to anterior half outer lip of iliac crest. Aponeurosis inserts medially to linea alba and inferiorly to pubic symphysis crest and tubercle. From ASIS to pubic tubercle forms the inguinal ligament and lacunar ligament. Posterior border lies free	Ventral rami of lowest six thoracic nerves	Raise intra-abdominal pressure, defaecation, micturition, parturition ⎫⎪⎬ Flexion and lateral flexion of spine ⎪⎭ Assist with expiration
Obliquus internus abdominis (internal oblique)	Lateral two-thirds of inguinal ligament. Anterior two-thirds of the intermediate line of iliac crest. Thoracolumbar fascia	Inferior fibres: Pubic crest and pectineal line as conjoint tendon. Aponeurosis forms medially and diverges: Upper part is attached to costal cartilages of 7th–9th ribs. Central part divides into two lamellae around rectus abdominis which join medially and insert into linea alba (1 cm below unbilicus aponeurosis runs anterior to rectus only). Posterior part to inferior borders of	Ventral rami of lowest six thoracic nerves L1	

Myology 147

Muscle	Origin	Insertion	Nerve supply	Action
Cremaster	Fibres of transversus abdominus and internal oblique from inguinal ligament	Form spiral loops attached to cord and tunica vaginalis which return to attach to pubic tubercle	Genital branch of genitofemoral N. L1,2	Pulls testis towards superficial inguinal ring
Transversus abdominus	Lateral one-third inguinal ligament Anterior two-thirds inner surface of lip of iliac crest Thoracolumbar fascia from iliac crest to 12th rib Internal surfaces of lower six costal cartilages interdigitating with fibres of diaphragm	Aponeurosis forms medially: Inserts into linea alba; upper three-quarters runs posterior and lower one-quarter anterior to rectus abdominis Inferior fibres form conjoint tendon	Ventral rami lower six thoracic and L1 spinal nerves	Acts with external internal oblique muscles
		lower four ribs, interdigitating with internal intercostal muscles		
Rectus abdominis (two heads)	*Lateral head:* Pubic crest *Medial head:* symphysis pubis interdigitating with opposite side	Three slips to external surfaces of costal cartilages 5th, 6th and 7th ribs	Ventral rami of lower six to seven thoracic nerves	Acts with oblique muscles On their own flex the trunk
Pyramidalis	Front of pubis and symphysis	Linea alba midway between umbilicus and symphysis	Subcostal nerve T12	Tense rectus sheath
Quadratus lumborum	Iliolumbar ligament and adjacent iliac crest	Medial half lower border 12th rib. Tips of TPs L1–L4	T12–L4 segmental nerves	Fixes 12th rib Extension and lateral flexion of lumbar spine

MUSCLES OF THE PELVIS

Muscle	Origin	Insertion	Nerve supply	Action
Levator ani (Divided into iliococcygeus and pubococcygeus)	Pelvic surface of body of pubis. 'White line' of obturator fascia. Medial surface of ischial spine	Most anterior fibres into perineal body (levator prostatae in men, sphincter vaginae in women) Intermediate fibres sling around rectum (puborectalis) Posterior fibres attach to coccyx and midline raphe between coccyx and anorectal junction	Branch of S4 Branches from inferior rectal nerve and perineal division of pudendal nerve	Support of pelvic floor. Maintenance of continence
Coccygeus	Medial surface of ischial spine and sacrospinous ligament	Coccyx and lowest piece of sacrum	Branches of S4, S5	Supports coccyx in defaecation

MUSCLES OF THE PERINEUM

Muscle	Origin	Insertion	Nerve supply	Action
Transverse perinei superficialis	Ischial tuberosity	Perineal body with its opposite partner	perineal branch of pudendal nerve S2, S3, S4	Fix perineal body
Bulbospongiosus	Perineal body anteriorly and median raphe	*Male*: Posterior fibres: perineal membrane Middle fibres: clasp corpus spongiosum and bulb of penis Anterior fibres: clasp corpus cavernosum and insert into radial aspect of penis *Female*: surrounds vagina; corpora cavernosa clitoridis		Empty urethra Assist in ejaculation Maintain erection Erection of clitoris
Ischiocavernosus	Ramus of ischium Tuberosity of ischium	*Male*: sides and under surface of crus of penis *Female*: Crura of clitoris		Maintenance of erection Erection of clitoris
Transverse perinei profundus	Ramus of ischium	Perineal body to meet opposite partner		Fix perineal body
Sphincter urethrae	Superficial fibres: pubic ramus Deep fibres: encircle membranous urethra	Perineal body		Compress and empty membranous urethra Assists in ejaculation in the male

MUSCLES OF THE UPPER LIMB

Muscles connecting upper limb to vertebral column and thoracic wall

Muscle	Origin	Insertion	Nerve supply	Action
Trapezius	Medial one-third superior nuchal line External occipital protuberance Ligamentum nuchae; spinous processes and supraspinous ligaments C6–T12	Posterior border lateral one-third of clavicle. Medial edge of acromion; crest of spine of scapula	*Motor*: accessory nerve (CX1) *Sensory*: cervical plexus C3, C4	Stability of scapula Movement of scapula protraction retraction elevation rotation
Latissimus dorsi	Spines of T7–T12; thoracolumbar fascia; crest of ilium Lower three to four ribs, interdigitating with external oblique	Bicipital groove of humerus	Thoracodorsal nerve C6, C7, C8	Extension, adduction and medial rotation of humerus Accessory muscle of respiration
Serratus anterior	Outer, superior surfaces of ribs 1st–8th. Lower four slips interdigitate with external oblique	Superior angle, costal surface of medial edge and inferior angle of scapula	Long thoracic nerve (of Bell) C5, C6, C7	Protraction and rotation of scapula Stability of scapula
Rhomboideus major	Vertebral spines and supraspinous ligaments T2–T5	Medial edge of blade of scapula	Dorsal scapular nerve C4, C5	Control position of scapula Retraction: rhomboids Rotation of scapula so glenoid fossa faces downwards
Rhomboideus minor	Vertebral spines C7, T1. Lower part of ligamentum nuchae	Medial edge of spine of scapula	Dorsal scapular nerve C4, C5	
Levator scapulae	Transverse processes C1–C4	Medial edge of scapula above spine	Segmental: C3, C4 spinal nerves C5 Dorsal scapular nerve	

Pectoralis major	Medial half clavicle; anterior surface of sternum Costal cartilages of 2nd–6th (occasionally 1st–7th) ribs Aponeurosis of external oblique	Bicipital groove of humerus	Lateral and medial pectoral nerves C(5), C6, C7, C8	Adduction and medial rotation of humerus Accessory muscle of respiration
Pectoralis minor	Upper, outer surfaces of 3rd–5th ribs	Coracoid process of scapula	Lateral and medial pectoral nerves C6, C7, C8	Protraction and rotation of scapula
Subclavius	Costochondral junction of 1st rib	Medial one-third inferior surface of clavicle	Branch from brachial plexus C5, C6	Stabilizes clavicle during shoulder movements
Deltoid	Lateral one-third clavicle Lateral and upper surface of acromion Crest of scapula spine	Deltoid tuberosity of humerus	Axillary nerve C5, C6	Whole muscle: abduction of humerus Anterior fibres: medial rotation Posterior fibres: lateral rotation
Subscapularis	Medial two-thirds of subscapular fossa	Lesser tuberosity of humerus	Upper and lower subscapular nerves C5, C6, (7)	Stabilizes head of humerus in shoulder joint, known collectively as the rotator cuff, with infraspinatus, supraspinatus and teres minor Individually on humerus: medial rotation of humerus
Supraspinatus	Medial two-thirds of supraspinous fossa	Greater tuberosity of humerus	Suprascapular nerves C5, C6	Initiation of abduction

Myology 151

Muscle	Origin	Insertion	Nerve supply	Action
Infraspinatus	Medial two-thirds of infraspinous fossa	Greater tuberosity of humerus	Suprascapular nerve C4, C5, C6	Medial rotation of humerus
Teres minor	Upper two-thirds of lateral posterior border of scapula	Greater tuberosity of humerus	Axillary nerve C5, C6	Lateral rotation and adduction of humerus
Teres major	Oval area at inferior angle on posterior surface of scapula	Bicipital groove of humerus	Lower subscapular nerve C6, C7	Adduction, medial rotation and extension of humerus

Muscles of upper arm

Muscle	Origin	Insertion	Nerve supply	Action
Coracobrachialis	Apex of coracoid process	Medial aspect of humeral shaft between origins of triceps and brachialis	Musculocutaneous nerve C5, C6, C7	Flexion and adduction of humerus
Biceps brachii (two heads)	*Short head:* apex of coracoid process *Long head:* supraglenoid tubercle	Tuberosity of radius and the deep fascia of forearm via the bicipital aponeurosis	Musculocutaneous nerve C5, C6	Supination of forearm Flexion of elbow (stability of humeral head in glenoid fossa)
Brachialis	Lower half anterior surface of humeral shaft; medial and lateral intermuscular septa	Tuberosity of ulna Coronoid process	Musculocutaneous nerve C5, C6 Lateral part of muscle: radial nerve C7	Flexion of elbow

Triceps (three heads)	*Long head:* infraglenoid tubercle *Lateral head:* ridge on posterior surface of humerus; lateral border of humerus *Medial head:* posterior surface of humeral shaft below spiral groove. Medial aspect of shaft. Medial and lower part of lateral intermuscular septa	Posterior aspect of olecranon Few fibres to capsule of elbow joint	Radial nerve C6, C7, C8	Extension of elbow Supports inferior aspect of humeral head

Muscles of the forearm

Common flexor origin (CFO): tendinous attachment to medial epicondyle of humerus

Pronator teres (two heads)	*Humeral head:* humerus above medial epicondyle and CFO *Ulna head:* medial side of coronoid process	Lateral aspect of shaft of radius	Median nerve C6, C7	Pronation of forearm (flexion of elbow)
Flexor carpi radialis (FCR)	CFO	Palmar surface, bases of 2nd and 3rd metacarpals	Median nerve C6, C7	Flexion of wrist with FCU Abduction of wrist with radial extensors
Palmaris longus	CFO	Palmar aponeurosis with slip to thenar muscles	Median nerve C8	Flexion of wrist

Muscle	Origin	Insertion	Nerve supply	Action
Flexor carpi ulnaris (FCU) (two heads)	*Humeral head*: CFO *Ulnar head*: medial edge of olecranon and upper two-thirds of posterior border of ulna via aponeurosis	Pisiform Hamate and 5th metacarpal via the pisohamate and pisometacarpal ligaments	Ulnar nerve C8, T1	Flexion of wrist with FCR Adduction of wrists with ECU
Flexor digitorum superficialis (two heads)	*Humero-ulnar head*: CFO: medial ligament of elbow. Medial aspect of coronoid process *Radial head*: Anterior surface of radius between radial tuberosity and insertion of pronator teres	Four tendons to the four fingers. Each inserts into the shaft of the middle phalanx after tendon separates for the passage of tendon of flexor digitorum profundus	Median nerve C7, C8, T1	Flexion of middle and proximal phalanges Flexion of wrist
Flexor digitorum profundus	Upper three-quarters of anterior and medial surface of ulna Medial aspect of coronoid process	Base of palmar surfaces of distal phalanges of all four fingers	Medial part via ulnar nerve. Lateral part via anterior interosseous nerve	Flexion of distal phalanges
Flexor pollicis longus	Anterior surface of radius below tuberosity Adjacent interosseous membrane	Palmar surface base of distal phalanx of thumb	Anterior interosseous nerve C8, T1	Flexion of phalanges of thumb
Pronator quadratus	Oblique ridge on lower anterior surface of ulna Lower one-quarter of medial surface of ulna	Lower one-quarter of anterior surface of radius	Anterior interosseous nerve C8, T1	Pronation of forearm Prevents separation of ulna and radius

Myology 155

Common extensor origin (CEO): tendinous attachment to front of lateral epicondyle of humerus

Brachioradialis	Upper two-thirds lateral supracondylar ridge of humerus. Anterior aspect of adjacent lateral intermuscular septum	Lateral aspect of radius just proximal to styloid process	Radial nerve C5, C6 (7)	Flexion of elbow
Extensor carpi radialis longus (ECRL)	Lower one-third lateral supracondylar ridge of humerus Lateral intermuscular septum	Radial side, dorsal surface of the base of 2nd metacarpal	Radial nerve C6, C7	Extension of wrist with ECRB and ECU Abduction of wrist with FCR
Extensor carpi radialis brevis (ECRB)	CEO Lateral ligament of elbow joint	Dorsal surfaces of bases 3rd and adjacent 2nd metacarpals	Posterior interosseous nerve C7, C8	As above
Extensor digitorum	CEO	Four tendons one to each finger blending with the dorsal digital expansion. Distally divides into two collateral slips and a central intermediate slip. Central slip to base of middle phalanx. Collateral slips unite distally to insert into base of distal phalanx	Posterior interosseous nerve C7, C8	Extension of finger at MCPJ and IPJ. Extension of wrist

Muscle	Origin	Insertion	Nerve supply	Action
Extensor digiti minimi	CEO	Dorsal extensor apparatus of little finger	Posterior interosseous nerve C7, C8	Extension of little finger
Extensor carpi ulnaris (ECU)	CEO Posterior surface of ulna via aponeurosis	Tubercle on ulna side of base of 5th metacarpal	Posterior interosseous nerve C7, C8	Extension of wrist with ECRL and ECRB Adduction of wrist with FCU
Anconeus	Posterior surface of lateral epicondyle of humerus	Lateral aspect of olecranon Upper posterior surface of ulna	Radial nerve C7, C8	Extension of elbow
Supinator (two heads)	Superficial and deep with common origins: CEO; lateral ligament of elbow joint; annular ligament of superior radio-ulna joint; supinator crest of ulna	Lateral surface of proximal one-quarter of radius	Posterior interosseous nerve C5, C6	Supination of forearm
Abductor pollicis longus (APL)	Posterior surface of ulna, below anconeus; Interosseous membrane Middle one-third posterior surface of radius	Radial side base of 1st metacarpal and the trapezium	Posterior interosseous nerve C7, 8	Abduction of thumb Extension of thumb with EPL and EPB

Myology 157

Muscle	Origin	Insertion	Nerve supply	Action
Extensor pollicis brevis (EPB)	Posterior surface of shaft of radius, below APL Interosseous membrane	Dorsal surface base of proximal phalanx of thumb	Posterior interosseous nerve C7, C8	Extension of proximal phalanx of thumb
Extensor pollicis longus (EPL)	Middle one-third posterior surface of ulna below APL Interosseous membrane	Dorsal surface base of distal phalanx of thumb. Tendon receives slips from, APB laterally, from Add P medially	Posterior interosseous nerve C7, C8	Extension of distal phalanx of thumb; with EPB and APL extends proximal phalanx and 1st metacarpal of thumb
Extensor indicis	Posterior surface of ulna below EPL Interosseous membrane	Joins ulna side of tendon of extensor digitorum to index finger, to insert into extensor apparatus	Posterior interosseous nerve C7, C8	Extension of index finger

Muscles of the hand

Muscle	Origin	Insertion	Nerve supply	Action
Abductor pollicis brevis (APB)	Flexor retinaculum and a few fibres from tubercles of scaphoid and trapezium	Medial fibres to radial side base of proximal phalanx Lateral fibres to dorsal expansion of thumb	Lateral terminal branch of median nerve C8, T1	Adduction and medial rotation of thumb
Opponens pollicis (OP)	Tubercle of trapezium Flexor retinaculum	Lateral border of 1st metacarpal	As above	Flexion and medial rotation of 1st metacarpal
Flexor pollicis brevis (FPB) (two parts)	*Superficial part:* Tubercle of trapezium and flexor retinaculum *Deep part:* trapezoid and capitate bones	Radial side base of proximal phalanx of thumb	Terminal branch median nerve and deep branch ulnar nerve C8, T1	Flexion of proximal phalanx. Flexion and medial rotation of 1st metacarpal with OP

Muscle	Origin	Insertion	Nerve supply	Action
Adductor pollicis (Add P) (two heads)	*Oblique head:* Capitate and bases 2nd and 3rd metacarpals *Transverse head:* Distal two-third of palmar surface of 3rd metacarpal	Two heads unite prior to insertion. Sesamoid bone in tendon. Ulnar border of base of proximal phalanx of thumb. Slip to dorsal expansion of thumb. Slip to FPB	Deep branch ulnar nerve C8, T1	Adduction of thumb
Palmaris brevis	Flexor retinaculum and palmar aponeurosis	Skin over ulna border of hand	Superficial branch of ulnar nerve C8, T1	Deepens hollow of palm
Abductor digiti minimi (ADM)	Pisiform bone; tendon of FCU; pisohamate ligament	Two slips to little finger: Ulnar side base of proximal phalanx Ulnar side of dorsal digital expansion	Deep branch ulnar nerve C8, T1	Abducts little finger from 4th finger
Flexor digiti minimi (FDM)	Hook of hamate Flexor retinaculum	Ulnar side, base of proximal phalanx of little finger	As above	Flexion of proximal phalanx
Opponens digiti minimi	Hook of hamate Flexor retinaculum	Ulnar border of 5th metacarpal	As above	Deepens hollow of palm by rotating metacarpal laterally
Lumbricals	Tendons of flexor digitorum profundus 1st and 2nd *(unipennate):* Radial side of tendons to index and middle	Radial side lateral aspect of dorsal extensor apparatus of same finger	1st and 2nd: Median nerve C8 T1	Flexion of MCPJ Extension of IPJ

Myology 159

Interossei (two groups)	*Dorsal group (bipennate):* Four dorsal muscles arise from adjacent sides of metacarpals, e.g. 1st dorsal interosseous from medial side of 1st metacarpal and lateral side of 2nd metacarpal	Dorsal extensor apparatus and bases of proximal phalanx of: 1st: radial side of index finger 2nd: radial side of middle finger 3rd: ulnar side of middle finger 4th: ulnar side of ring finger	*3rd and 4th:* Deep branch ulnar nerve C8 T1	*3rd and 4th (bipennate):* Adjacent sides of tendons to middle and ring (3rd); ring and little (4th) fingers Abducts fingers away from middle finger
	Palmar group (unipennate): palmar surfaces of: 1st: ulnar side of 1st metacarpal 2nd: ulnar surface of 2nd metacarpal 3rd: radial side of 4th metacarpal 4th: radial side of 5th metacarpal	Base of proximal phalanx and dorsal extensor apparatus of: 1st: ulnar border of thumb 2nd: ulnar border index finger 3rd: radial border ring finger 4th: radial border little finger	Deep branch ulnar nerve C8, T1	Adduct fingers towards middle finger

MUSCLES OF THE LOWER LIMB

Muscles of the iliac region

Muscle	Origin	Insertion	Nerve supply	Action
Psoas Major	Transverse processes of lumbar vertebrae. Five slips, each arising from an intervertebral disc and adjacent vertebral bodies and tendinous arches which stretch across each vertebral body T12–L5	Lesser trochanter of femur	Ventral rami of lumbar nerves L1, L2, L3	In combination with iliacus Flexion of hip, medial rotation of femur
Psoas Minor	Side of bodies T12–L1 and the intervertebral disc	Iliopectineal eminence	Branch of 1st lumbar nerve	Flexor of trunk
Iliacus	Upper two-thirds of iliac fossa; Inner lip of iliac crest; Anterior sacroiliac and iliolumbar ligaments; Lateral part of sacrum	Lateral aspect of psoas tendon	Femoral nerve L2, L3	With Psoas major flexion of hip and medial rotation of femur

Muscles of thigh and gluteal region

Tensor fasciae lata	Anterior 5 cm outer lip of iliac crest Anterior superior iliac spine. Deep surface of fascia lata	Iliotibial tract	Superior gluteal nerve L4, L5	Assists in steadying pelvis on femur and in steadying condyles of femur on tibia. Important in maintaining erect posture
Sartorius	Anterior superior iliac spine and notch beneath	Upper part medial surface of tibia	Femoral nerve L2, L3	Flexion, abduction and lateral rotation of femur
Quadriceps femoris (Four parts forming anterior muscle of the leg)				
Rectus femoris (two heads)	*Straight head:* anterior inferior iliac spine *Reflected head:* groove above acetabulum	Quadriceps tendon is the union of all four muscles attached to the base of the patella. Patella is a sesamoid bone in the tendon. The 'Ligamentum' patella is the continuation of the quadriceps tendon from the apex of the patella inserted into the tubercle of the tibia. Some parts of the quadriceps tendon pass directly over the patella to the insertion	Femoral nerve L2, L3, L4	Extension of knee Flexion of hip
Vastus lateralis	Upper part of trochanteric line Anterior and inferior borders of greater trochanter Gluteal tuberosity Upper half lateral lip of linea aspera			

Muscle	Origin	Insertion	Nerve supply	Action
Vastus medialis	Lower part intertrochanteric line Spiral line Medial lip linea aspera Upper part medial supracondylar line Tendons of adductor longus and magnus Medial intermuscular septum	Expansion medially to capsule of knee joint and medial aspect of tibial condyle		Lower fibres maintain patella in its groove during extension of knee
Vastus intermedius	Anterior and lateral upper two-thirds of shaft of femur Lateral intermuscular septum			
Articularis genu	Lower anterior surface of shaft of femur	Synovial membrane of knee superiorly		Pulls synovium superiorly during extension
Gracilis	Medial margin body of pubis; inferior pubic ramus and adjoining ischial ramus	Upper part medial surface of tibia below condyle	Obturator nerve L2, L3	Flexes and adducts the leg Medial rotation of femur
Pectineus	Pectineal line of pubis	Line from lesser trochanter to linea aspera	Femoral nerve L2, L3	Flexion and adduction of the femur
Adductor longus	Pubis between crest and symphysis	Middle one-third of linea aspera between vastus lateralis and adductor magnus	Anterior division obturator nerve L2, L3, L4	Adduction of femur Maintenance of erect posture

Muscle	Origin	Insertion	Nerve	Action
Adductor brevis	External surface body and inferior ramus of pubis between gracilis and obturator externus	Line from lesser trochanter to linea aspera behind pectineus and adductor longus	Obturator Nerve L2, L3, L4	As above
Adductor magnus	Inferior ramus of pubis	Medial margin of gluteal tuberosity of femur	Obturator nerve L3, L4	As above
	Ramus of ischium	Linea aspera and upper part medial supracondylar line		
	Inferior part of ischial tuberosity	Adductor tubercle of femur	Tibial division of sciatic nerve L2, L3, L4	As above. Also weak extensor of thigh
Gluteus maximus	Posterior gluteal line of ilium	Superficial part to iliotibial tract	Inferior gluteal nerve L5, S1, S2	Maintaining erect attitude of body. Abduction and extension of the hip
	Rough part of ilium and crest, above and behind posterior gluteal line	Deep part into gluteal tuberosity		
	Aponeurosis of sacrospinalis			
	Posterior surface of lower sacrum and coccyx			
	Sacrotuberous ligament			
	Fascia over gluteus medius			
Gluteus medius	Outer surface of ilium between, posterior gluteal line and iliac crest superiorly, and middle gluteal line inferiorly	Greater trochanter	Superior gluteal nerve L5, S1	Abduction medial rotation of femur Important in posture and gait

Muscle	Origin	Insertion	Nerve supply	Action
Gluteus minimus	Outer surface of ilium between middle and inferior gluteal lines Margin of greater sciatic notch	Greater trochanter	Superior gluteal nerve L5, S1	As above
Piriformis	Pelvic surface of sacrum by three slips from area of bone between anterior sacral foramina	Greater trochanter	Branches from L5, S1, S2	Lateral rotation of extended thigh Abducts flexed thigh
Obturator internus	Inner surface of anterolateral wall of the pelvis, surrounding the obturator foramen. Attached to inferior pubic ramus, ischial ramus, pelvic surface of ilium, medial part of obturator membrane and tendinous arch over obturator canal	Medial surface of greater trochanter	Nerve to obturator internus L5, S1	Lateral rotation of extended thigh Abducts flexed thigh
Superior gemellus	Posterior surface of ischial spine	Tendon of obturator internus	Nerve to obturator internus L5, S1	As above
Inferior gemellus	Ischial tuberosity	Lower part of obturator internus tendon	Nerve to quadratus femoris L5, S1	As above
Quadratus femoris	Upper part of outer surface of ischial tuberosity	Tubercle on upper part of trochanteric crest and small part of bone beneath it	Nerve to quadratus femoris L5, S1	Lateral rotation of thigh

Muscle	Origin	Insertion	Nerve supply	Action
Obturator externus	Outer surface of pelvis around medial margin of obturator foramen. Attached to ramus of pubis, ischium and outer surface of obturator membrane	Trochanteric fossa of femur	Posterior division obturator nerve L3, L4	As above
Biceps femoris (two heads)	*Long head:* Ischial tuberosity and sacrotuberous ligament *Short head:* Linea aspera Lateral supracondylar line Lateral intermuscular septum	Head of fibula; slips to fibula collateral ligament and lateral tibial condyle	Sciatic nerve Long head via tibial part and short head via common peroneal part L5, S1, S2	Flex leg on thigh Maintenance of upright posture Extends hip from below
Semitendinosus	Ischial tuberosity in common with biceps femoris	Upper part medial surface of tibial shaft	Sciatic nerve (tibial part) L5, S1, S2	As above
Semimembranosus	Ischial tuberosity and ramus. Fibres linked with biceps femoris and semitendinosus	Groove on posterior aspect of medial tibial condyle Expansion to form oblique posterior ligament of knee	Sciatic nerve (tibial) L5, S1, S2	As above

Muscles of the leg

Muscle	Origin	Insertion	Nerve supply	Action
Tibialis anterior	Lateral tibial condyle, upper two-thirds of lateral surface shaft of tibia, anterior surface interosseous membrane and intermuscular septum	Medial cuneiform and base of 1st metatarsal	Deep peroneal nerve L4, L5	Dorsiflexion of the ankle and invertor of foot. Maintains longitudinal arch of foot
Extensor hallucis longus	Middle two-thirds of anterior surface fibula. Anterior surface interosseous membrane	Dorsal aspect base of distal phalanx of the great toe	Deep peroneal nerve L5, S1	Extension of great toe. Dorsiflexion of ankle
Extensor digitorum longus	Lateral condyle of tibia. Upper three-quarters of medial surface of shaft of fibula. Anterior surface of interosseous membrane and intermuscular septum	Divides into four tendons over dorsum of foot and inserts into dorsal digital expansion as in the hand	Deep peroneal nerve L5, S1	Extends toes. Dorsiflexion of ankle

Peroneus tertius	Lower one-quarter of medial surface of shaft fibula Interosseous membrane	Dorsal surface base of 5th of metatarsal	As above	Dorsiflexion and eversion of foot
Peroneus longus	Head and upper two-thirds of lateral surface shaft of fibula; adjacent intermuscular septa	Two slips into lateral side of base of 1st metatarsal and lateral side of medial cuneiform. Tendon passes obliquely across sole of foot from lateral to medial	Superficial peroneal nerve L5, S1, S2	Eversion and dorsiflexion of foot Maintenance of upright posture
Peroneus brevis	Lower two-thirds of lateral surface shaft of fibula. Intermuscular septa	Tubercle on lateral side base 5th metatarsal	Superficial peroneal nerve L5, S1, S2	Eversion of foot Maintenance of upright posture
Gastrocnemius (two heads)	*Medial*: upper and posterior part of medial femoral condyle. Popliteal surface of femur *Lateral*: lateral surface of lateral femoral condyle and lower part lateral supracondylar line	United with tendon of soleus to form tendo achilles to insert into posterior surface of calcaneus	Tibial nerve S1, S2	Plantar flexion of foot

Muscle	Origin	Insertion	Nerve supply	Action
Soleus	Posterior surface of head and upper quarter of shaft of fibula. Soleal line and middle one-third of medial border of tibia with fibrous arch between fibula and tibia	Via tendo achilles into posterior surface of calcaneus	Tibial nerve S1, S2	Plantar flexion and maintenance of upright posture
Plantaris	Lateral supracondylar line of femur and oblique popliteal ligament	Posterior surface of calcaneus	Tibial nerve S1, S2	With gastrocnemius
Popliteus	Tendinous origin from lateral condyle of femur and arcuate popliteal ligament and lateral meniscus	Triangular area above soleal line of posterior surface of tibia	Tibial nerve L4, L5, S1	Rotation of tibia medially on femur Draws meniscus backwards during flexion of knee
Flexor hallucis longus	Inferior two-thirds of posterior surface of shaft of fibula Posterior surface interosseous membrane and intermuscular septa	Plantar surface base of distal phalanx of great toe	Tibial nerve S2, S3	Flexion of toes. Maintenance of upright posture
Flexor digitorum longus (FDL)	Posterior surface of shaft of tibia below soleal line	Divides into four tendons in the foot Each inserts into plantar surface of distal phalanges of 2nd–5th toes	Tibial nerve S2, S3	As above

Tibialis posterior	Posterior surface of interosseous membrane Lateral aspect posterior surface of tibia below soleal line Upper two-thirds of posterior aspect of shaft of fibula. Intermuscular septa	Tuberosity of navicular and via slips to: sustentaculum tali, bases of 2nd–4th metatarsals, and cuneiform bones	Tibial nerve L4, L5	Inversion of foot Maintenance of longitudinal arch Maintenance of upright posture

Muscles of the foot

Extensor digitorum brevis	Anterior part of superolateral surface of calcaneus Talocalcaneal ligaments and inferior extensor retinaculum	Four tendons insert into lateral sides of tendons of EDL 2nd–4th toes, and base of proximal phalanx of great toe	Lateral terminal branch of deep peroneal nerve S1, S2	Extension of toes

Plantar muscles: first layer

Abductor hallucis	Medial tubercle of calcaneus and plantar aponeurosis	Medial side base of proximal phalanx of great toe	Medial plantar nerve S2, S3	Precise details of the function of the intrinsic muscles are unknown. They most probably act to give the best construction of the foot for standing and walking

Muscle	Origin	Insertion	Nerve supply	Action
Flexor digitorum brevis	Medial tubercle of calcaneus and plantar aponeurosis	Four tendons to middle phalanges of 2nd–5th toes. Divides to allow passage of tendons of FDL	Medial plantar nerve S2, S3	
Abductor digiti minimi	Lateral and medial tubercles of calcaneus. Plantar aponeurosis	Lateral side base of proximal phalanx 5th toe	Lateral plantar nerve S2, S3	
Second layer				
Flexor digitorum accessorius (two heads)	*Medial*: medial concave surface of calcaneus. *Lateral*: calcaneus in front of lateral tubercle and long plantar ligament	Lateral border of tendon of FDL	Lateral plantar nerve S2, S3	
Lumbricals (four)	Arise from adjacent tendons of FDL. 1st only one slip from medial aspect tendon FDL to 2nd toe	Dorsal digital expansions on medial sides of four lesser toes	1st: medial plantar nerve 2nd–4th: deep branch of lateral plantar nerve S2, S3	
Third layer				
Flexor hallucis brevis	Y-shaped origin. *Lateral limb*: medial part plantar surface of cuboid and adjacent lateral cuneiform. *Medial limb*: Tibialis posterior tendon	Inserts as two slips into either side base of proximal phalanx of great toe	Medial plantar nerve S2, S3	

Muscle	Origin	Insertion	Nerve supply
Adductor hallucis (two heads)	*Oblique*: Bases of 2nd–4th metatarsals *Transverse*: Plantar metatarsophalangeal ligaments of 3rd–5th toes. Deep transverse metatarsal ligaments	Lateral side base of proximal phalanx of great toe	Deep branch of lateral plantar nerve of S2, S3
Flexor digiti minimi brevis	Medial part plantar surface of 5th metatarsal	Lateral side base of proximal phalanx of 5th toe	Superficial branch of lateral plantar nerve S2, S3
Fourth layer			
Interossei (two heads)	*Dorsal*: four bipennate muscles from adjacent sides of metatarsal shafts, e.g. 1st from 1st and 2nd metatarsal shafts	1st medial aspect dorsal digital expansion and base of proximal phalanx of 2nd toe 2nd–4th lateral aspect of dorsal digital expansion and base of proximal phalanges of 3rd–5th toes	Deep branch of lateral plantar nerve except 4th space which is supplied by superficial branch S2, S3
	Plantar: three unipennate muscles from bases and medial surfaces of 3rd–5th metatarsal shafts	Medial sides dorsal digital expansion and bases of proximal phalanges 3rd–5th toes	

Myology 171

ARTHROLOGY

CLASSIFICATION OF JOINTS
Joints are classified as:
1. Fibrous joints: synarthroses (fixed)
2. Cartilaginous joints: amphiarthroses (slightly movable)
3. Synovial joints: diarthroses (freely movable)

FIBROUS AND CARTILAGINOUS JOINTS

Synchrondoses
Temporary cartilaginous junction between a diaphysis and epiphysis during growth. Regions of unossified cartilage between growing bones in the skull.

Sutures
Limited to the skull, occurring where two bones meet and articulate and separated by connective tissue called the sutural ligament. These sutural ligaments ossify in later life.

Schindylesis
Articulation where a ridged bone fits into a groove, e.g. vomer and sphenoid.

Gomphosis
Fixation of teeth into mandible as a peg and socket arrangement.

Syndesmosis
Where two loosely-linked bones are held together by an interosseous ligament. Includes interosseus membranes in the forearm and leg. The inferior tibio fibular joint is considered a syndesmosis.

Symphysis
Fibrocartilaginous articulation with no synovium or capsule. Limited range of movement, all lie in the median plane of the body. All parts are united there are no internal surfaces.

The terms primary and secondary cartilaginous joints are no longer in use: primary cartilaginous refers to synchondroses while secondary cartilaginous refers to symphyses.

SYNOVIAL JOINTS

Structure
1. Fibrous capsule, enclose the joint completely with few exceptions
2. Synovial membrane. Lines the capsule and all intra-articular structures except discs of fibrocartilage or menisci
3. Articular surface: hyaline cartilage designed for the high wear, low friction and high forces necessary for joint movement
4. Synovial fluid: non-Newtonian fluid, it is a dialysate of plasma. It acts to lubricate the joint and provide nutrition for the articular surfaces

Classification

Complexity of organization
1. Simple joints: two surfaces
2. Compound joint: more than two surfaces
3. Complex joint: presence of intra-articular disc or cartilage

Morphological classication
1. Plane joint: apposition of flat articular surfaces
2. Hinge joint: uniaxial with strong collateral ligaments
3. Pivot joint: uniaxial with rotation about a long axis
4. Bicondylar: principle movement in one direction with slight movement in another at 90° to the first
5. Ellipsoid: biaxial with two planes of movement
6. Sellar (saddle) joint: biaxial; movement in two planes is accompanied by rotation in a long axis
7. Spheroidal (ball-and-socket) joints: multiaxial

Movements of joints
1. Translation: sliding movement
2. Angular movement:
   a. flexion and extension, i.e. bending and straightening occur about a transverse axis
   b. abduction and adduction occur around an anteroposterior axis.
3. Circumduction: compound movement of flexion, extension, abduction and adduction
4. Rotation: movement about a longitudinal axis

Some joints do provide exception to the above.

Blood supply
Branches of periarticular plexi pierce capsule to form a vascular plexus in the synovial membrane

Lymphatic drainage
Lymphatic plexi in the synovium drain to regional lymph nodes

Nerve supply
General rule: nerves of muscles acting on a joint also innervate the joint (Hiltons law).

Capsule has a rich nerve supply involved in the sensations of pain, stretch, position and vibration. Specialized sensory endings register speed and direction of movement. Synovium has relatively little nerve supply.

OSTEOLOGY

BONE

The human skeleton is an endoskeleton, i.e. internal to the muscles. The individual bones vary in shape and size and can be classified into long, short, flat and irregular.
1. Long bones
   a. tubular structures with central medullary cavity
   b. expanded ends for articulation
   c. often multiple epiphyses and ossification centres
2. Short bones: thin external shell of compact bone supported by an interior of trabecular bone
3. Flat bones: middle layer of trabecular bone enclosed between two laminae of compact bone
4. Irregular bones: no particular structure.

STRUCTURE OF MATURE BONE

Macroscopic
Compact bone on the exterior with trabecular (cancellous, spongy) bone on the interior. The thickness and exact composition varies between individual bones. In the tubular long bones the central medullary cavity is filled with bone marrow, either haemopoetic or adipose. The external surface of bone is covered by a fibrous layer, the periosteum, except over articular surfaces which are covered by articular cartilage.

Microscopic
1. Compact bone: haversian system of cylindrical units (secondary osteons) which vary in size and orientation, usually longitudinal and consist of:
   a. central haversian canal containing a neurovascular bundle surrounded by concentric lamellae of bone. Between lamellae are lacunae, spaces containing osteocytes. Lacunae and central canal are interconnected by a fine network of canaliculi

b. interstitial bone fills the space between the cylinders. Lamellae arranged in various directions
The outer surface of the bone may be formed by circumferential lamellae surrounding the cylindrical units.
2. Trabecular bone: irregular structure of lamellae which do not have a haversian system. Nutrition is direct from surrounding marrow vessels
3. Lamella: plate of bony tissue made up of a ground substance (matrix) with collagen fibres and mineral salt deposition
Uncalcified matrix is called osteoid.

GROWTH IN BONE

Bones are pre-formed in soft tissue, either hyaline cartilage (cartilaginous) or condensed mesenchyme (membranous). Ossification occurs from ossification centres; some bones have a single centre, e.g. carpal bones, while others, particularly long bones, have a primary centre which appears in utero (IU) with secondary centres that appear during childhood. Thus long bones are divided into:
1. Diaphysis (shaft): ossified from the primary centre
2. Epiphysis: the end of a long bone. Ossified from a secondary centre
3. Metaphysis: the part of the diaphysis adjacent to the growth plate where active growth occurs

The diaphysis and epiphysis are separated by the growth plate (epiphysial plate). This is a disc of cartilage where longitudinal growth occurs. Growth ceases when fusion of the diaphysis and epiphysis occurs across the plate and the bone is a single ossified unit. Epiphyses may be single or multiple, occur at one end or both.

BLOOD SUPPLY

1. Long bones
   a. arterial supply
      (i) one to two diaphyseal nutrient arteries
      (ii) metaphyseal vessels from nearby systemic arteries
      (iii) epiphyseal vessels from periarticular network of vessels
   b. venous drainage: vessels that leave from the entire surface of the bone to nearest systemic vein
2. Short, flat and irregular bones: these receive their blood supply direct from the overlying periosteum and the larger irregular bones may also have nutrient vessels

LYMPHATIC DRAINAGE

Vessels within the periosteum but not known to be in bone substance.

Osteology 177

NERVE SUPPLY
Myelinated and non-myelinated fibres accompany diaphyseal vessels.

OSSIFICATION
The times of appearance of primary and secondary centres of ossification, and the sequence and timing of fusion in individual bones are detailed below.

AXIAL SKELETON

Typical vertebra

Appearance
1. Primary centres (three)
   a. body: 3rd month IU (thoracic vertebrae first)
   b. each half of vertebral arch: 7th–8th week IU (cervical vertebrae first)
2. Secondary centres (five)
   a. tip of transverse process
   b. tip of spinous process
   c. upper and lower borders of vertebral bodies; shaped as annular discs

All appear at puberty.

Fusion
1. Primary centres
   a. two halves of vertebral arch unite posteriorly: 1 year (lumbar vertebrae first)
   b. body and vertebral arch fuse
      (i) 3rd year (cervical)
      (ii) 6th year (lumbar)
2. Secondary centres: all fuse with main mass of vertebra: 20th–25th years

Cervical vertebra

Appearance
Two additional centres for the costal processes: 6th month IU

Fusion
Costal processes fuse with main mass: 5th–6th year.

Lumbar vertebra

Appearance
Two additional centres for the mamillary processes: puberty

Fusion
Mamillary processes fuse with main mass: 25th year.

Atlas

Appearance
Three centres
1. Each half of lateral mass: 7th week IU
2. Anterior arch: 1 year

Fusion
1. Lateral masses fuse posteriorly: 3rd–4th year
2. Anterior arch fuses with lateral mass: 6th–8th year

Axis

Appearance
1. Primary centres (five)
   a. each half of vertebral arch: 7th week IU
   b. body: 4th–5th week IU
   c. each half of dens: 6th month IU (laterally placed)
2. Secondary centres
   a. annular disc on lower surface of body: 12th year
   b. tip of dens (odontoid): 2nd year

Fusion
1. Primary centres
   a. vertebral arches and body fuse as a typical vertebra
   b. two halves of dens: at birth
2. Secondary centres
   a. annular disc to vertebra: 20th–25th year
   b. tip of dens to rest of dens: 12th year (the entire dens may remain separate from the body until late in life)

Sacrum

Appearance
1. Primary centres
   a. vertebral elements (three centres)
      (i) body: 10th–20th week IU
      (ii) each half of vertebral arch: 10th–20th week IU
   b. costal elements: each side of sacral vertebra: 6th–8th month IU
2. Secondary centres: all appear at puberty
   a. vertebral elements
      (i) upper and lower borders of each body
      (ii) spinous tubercles
      (iii) transverse tubercles

b. costal elements at the lateral extremities of vertebrae
   (i) anterior and posterior in S1, S2
   (ii) anterior only for the rest.

Fusion
1. Primary centres
   a. each half of vertebral arch and its corresponding costal element fuse each side: 2nd–5th year
   b. body and vertebral arches fuse from below upwards and across midline: 8th year–puberty
2. Secondary centres: all fuse to main mass from above downwards: 15th–20th year.

Coccyx

Appearance
1. Primary centres
   a. first segment: 1st–4th year
   b. second segment: 5th–10th year
   c. third segment: 10th–15th year
   d. fourth segment: 14th–20th year
2. Secondary centres
   a. at each coccygeal cornu
   b. a pair of epiphyseal plates for each level

Fusion
Segments fuse with each other late in life. First to second at 30 yrs

Sternum

Formed by the union of two cartilaginous plates across the midline.

Appearance
1. Manubrium (one to three centres): 5th month IU
2. Body (four to eight centres): 4th–8th month IU
   Each level may have single or paired centres
3. Xiphoid (one centre): 3rd year

Fusion
1. Centres in the body fuse together from below upwards: puberty–25th year
2. Xiphoid fuses with body: 40th year

Ribs

Appearance
1. Primary centre: shaft (6th–7th ribs first): 8th week IU
2. Secondary centres: all appear at puberty
   a. head
   b. tubercle

1st rib has only one secondary centre, for the tubercle. 11th and 12th ribs have no tubercles.

Fusion
Secondary centres fuse with the shaft: 20th–25th year.

CRANIAL BONES

Mandible
Formed in fibromembrane

Appearance
1. Ossification centre: single centre near mental foramen: 6th week IU
2. Secondary cartilage: appears as the condylar cartilage which is replaced by bone by the 20th week IU. A small area of cartilage persists beneath the head until the 30th year. Cartilaginous nodules at symphysis menti ossify in 7th month IU

Fusion
1. Two halves of mandible unite at symphysis: 1–2 years
2. Growth and changes in shape achieved by remodelling

Hyoid
Formed from cartilages of the 2nd and 3rd arches.

Appearance
Six centres
1. Body has two centres: birth
2. Each greater cornu: 9th month IU (3rd arch)
3. Each lesser cornu: puberty (2nd arch)

Fusion
1. Greater cornua to body: 30 years
2. Lesser cornua to body: 30 years onwards

Occipital bone
Squamous part formed in membrane above and cartilage below the superior nuchal line.

Appearance
1. Membranous part has two centres either side of midline: 2nd month IU
2. Cartilaginous part has two centres: 7th week IU (fuse together rapidly)
3. Lateral part: single centre: 8th week IU
4. Basilar part: single centre: 6th week IU

Osteology 181

Fusion
1. Membranous and cartilaginous parts fuse: 3rd month IU
2. Lateral part fuses with rest: 2nd year
3. Basilar part fuses with rest: 6th year

Occipital bone joins with the sphenoid to form one bone between 18th and 25th year.

Sphenoid

Two parts; pre- and post-sphenoid, Pre-sphenoid part lies in front of tuberculum and the lesser wings attach to it. Post-sphenoid part lies behind tuberculum and greater wing attaches to it.

Appearance
1. Pre-sphenoid part (six centres)
    a. each lesser wing: 9th week IU
    b. two centres for the body: 10th week IU
    c. each sphenoidal concha: 5th month IU
2. Post-sphenoidal part (eight centres)
    a. root of each greater wing: 8th week IU. (rest of wing and lateral pterygoid plate formed in membrane)
    b. two centres for the body: 4th month IU (fuse together immediately)
    c. each medial pterygoid plate: 9th–10th week IU
    d. each lingula: 4th month IU (fuse with body immediately)

Fusion
1. Sphenoidal conchae fuse with ethmoid labyrinth: 4th year (fuses with sphenoid and palatine bones: puberty)
2. Medial pterygoid plate fuses with lateral pterygoid plate: 6th month IU
3. Pre- and postsphenoidal parts fuse: 8th month IU

At birth the sphenoid consists of three parts:
1. Body and lesser wings united as one.
2. Greater wing and pterygoid process form two lateral parts.

These fuse at: 1 year.
Sphenoid unites with occipital bone: 18th–25th year.

Temporal

Appearance
1. Squamous part; centre at root of zygomatic arch: 7th–8th week IU (formed in membrane)
2. Tympanic part; one centre; 3rd month IU (formed in membrane)
3. Petromastoid part; multiple centres: 5th month IU (formed in cartilage)

4. Styloid process (formed from cartilage of 2nd arch) has two centres
   a. proximal centre: 9th month IU
   b. distal centre: after birth

Fusion
1. Squamous and tympanic parts fuse at: 9th month IU
2. Petromastoid fuses with rest at: 1 year
3. Proximal centre of styloid process fuses at: 1 year
4. Distal centre of styloid process fuses: puberty

Parietal (formed in membrane)
1. Two centres: 7th week IU
2. Fuse together in utero: ossification is centrifugal

Frontal (formed in membrane)
1. Two centres; one at each superciliary arch: 8th week IU
2. At birth the two halves are separated by the metopic suture. This fuses from front to back: 2nd–8th year

Ethmoid (formed in cartilage)
1. Three centres
   a. perpendicular plate: 1 year
   b. each labyrinth: 4th–5th month IU
2. Fuse together: 2nd year

Inferior nasal concha
Single centre: 5th month IU

Lacrimal bone
Single centre: 12th week IU

Nasal bone
Single centre: 3rd month IU

Vomer
1. Two centres; one either side of midline: 8th week IU
2. Fuse together: 12th week IU

Maxilla
1. Three centres
   a. single centre for main mass: 6th week IU
   b. two centres for pre-maxilla (os incisura): 7th week IU
2. Fuse together by 3rd month IU

Palatine bone
Single centre in perpendicular plate: 8th week IU

Zygoma
Single centre: 8th week IU

UPPER LIMB
Scapula
Appearance
Eight centres:
1. Centre of body: 8th week IU
2. Centre of coracoid process: 1st year
3. Root of coracoid process: 12th year
4. Base of acromion: 14th year
5. Inferior angle: 15th year
6. Tip of acromion: 16th year
7. Medial border: 17th year
8. Glenoid rim: 14th year

Occasionally a separate centre for tip of coracoid process.

Fusion
1. Centre of coracoid fuses with root of coracoid: 15th year
2. Root of coracoid fuses to body: 14th–17th year
3. Rest of centres fuse to body by the 20th year

Clavicle
Formed in membrane. First of any bone to ossify

Appearance
1. Primary centres: medial and lateral: 5th–6th week IU
2. Secondary centre: sternal end: 18th–20th year

Fusion
1. Primary centres unite by 45th day IU
2. Secondary centre fuses with shaft: 18th–20th year

Humerus
Appearance
1. Primary centre: shaft: 8th week IU
2. Secondary centre
   a. head: birth
   b. greater tuberosity: 2nd year
   c. lesser tuberosity: 5th year
   d. capitulum: 1st year
   e. trochlea: 10th year
   f. lateral epicondyle: 12th year
   g. medial epicondyle: 5th year

Fusion
1. Head, greater and lesser tuberosities fuse together by 6th year then fuse as one with the shaft at 20th year.
2. Capitulum, trochlea and lateral epicondyle fuse together at puberty then fuse with shaft 14th–16th year
3. Medial epicondyle fuses with shaft: 20th year

Radius

Appearance
1. Primary centre: shaft: 8th week IU
2. Secondary centres
   a. Distal end: 1st–2nd year
   b. Proximal end: 4th year

Occasionally separate centre for tuberosity 14th year

Fusion
1. Proximal end fuses: 17th year
2. Distal end fuses: 20th year

Ulna

Appearance
1. Primary centre: Shaft: 8th week IU
2. Secondary centres
   a. head: 5th–6th year
   b. olecranon: 11th year

Fusion
1. Head fuses: 17th–18th year
2. Olecranon fuses: 14th–16th year

Carpal bones

Single centres for each bone. Order of ossification may vary.

Appearance, in common order
1. Capitate: 2nd month
2. Hamate: 2nd month
3. Triquetral: 3rd year
4. Lunate: 4th year
5. Scaphoid: 5th year
6. Trapezoid: 5th–6th year
7. Trapezium: 5th–6th year
8. Pisiform: 12th year

Metacarpal bones

Appearance
1. Primary centres: shaft: 8th–9th weeks IU
   a. 2nd and 3rd metacarpals first
   b. 1st metacarpal last
2. Secondary centres
   a. heads of 2nd–5th metacarpals: 2nd–3rd years
   b. base of 1st metacarpal: 2nd–3rd year

Fusion
Secondary centres fuse with shaft: 15th–18th years

Phalanges

Appearance
1. Primary centres: shaft:
   a. distal phalanx: 8th week IU
   b. proximal phalanx: 10th week IU
   c. middle phalanx: 11th week IU
2. Secondary centres
   a. bases of proximal phalanges: 6th–12th month
   b. bases of middle and distal phalanges: 6 months later

Fusion
Secondary centres fuse with shaft: 17th year

LOWER LIMB

Hip bone

Appearance
1. Primary centres
   a. ilium above greater sciatic notch: 8th–9th week IU
   b. body of ischium: 4th month IU
   c. superior pubic ramus: 4th month IU
2. Secondary centres, all appear at puberty
   a. iliac crest, two centres which fuse together immediately
   b. anterior superior iliac spine
   c. ischial tuberosity
   d. acetabulum, two centres:
      (i) between ilium and pubis.
      (ii) between ilium and ischium.
Pubic tubercle, crest and symphysis may have separate centres.

Fusion
1. Primary centres: body of ischium and superior pubic ramus: 7th year
2. Secondary centres: ilium and secondary centres fuse with rest to form one bone by 20th year

Femur

Appearance
1. Primary centre; shaft: 7th week IU
2. Secondary centres
   a. distal end: 9th month IU
   b. head: 1st year
   c. greater trochanter: 4th year
   d. lesser trochanter: 12th year

Fusion
1. Lesser trochanter to shaft: puberty
2. Greater trochanter to shaft: 14th year
3. Head to shaft: 14th–17th year
4. Distal end to shaft: 16th–18th year

Tibia

Appearance
1. Primary centre; shaft: 7th week IU
2. Secondary centres
   a. upper end: at birth
   b. lower end: 1st year
   c. tuberosity: 12th year

Fusion
1. Upper end and tuberosity fuse soon after centre for latter appears then fuse to shaft: 16th–18th year
2. Lower end to shaft: 15th–17th year

Patella
Multiple centres appear: 3rd–6th year. Coalesce rapidly.

Fibula

Appearance
1. Primary centre; shaft: 8th week IU
2. Secondary centres
   a. lower end: 1st year
   b. upper end: 3rd–4th year

Fusion
1. Lower end fuses: 15th–17th year
2. Upper end fuses: 17th–19th year

Tarsal bones
1. Calcaneum
   a. Appearance
      (i) primary centre: 3rd month IU
      (ii) secondary centre: Posterior epiphysis: 6th–8th year
   b. Fusion: fuse together: 14th–16th year
2. Talus
   a. single centre: 6th month IU
   b. occasionally centre for the tubercle which if remains separate forms os trigonum
3. Cuboid: 9th month IU
4. Lateral cuneiform: 1st year
5. Medial cuneiform: 2nd year
6. Intermediate cuneiform: 3rd year
7. Navicular: 3rd year

Metatarsal bones
Appearance
1. Primary centre; shaft: 8th–9th week IU
2. Secondary centres
   a. base of 1st metatarsal: 3rd year
   b. heads of 2nd–5th metatarsals: 3rd–4th year
   c. centre at base of 5th metatarsal for the tubercle

Fusion
Secondary centres fuse to shaft: 17th–20th year

Phalanges
Appearance
1. Primary centre: shaft:
   a. distal phalanx: 8th–9th week IU
   b. proximal phalanx: 12th–16th week IU
   c. middle phalanx: 16th week IU
2. Secondary centres: bases of phalanges: 2nd–8th year

Fusion
Secondary centres fuse with shafts: 17th–18th year

CRANIAL FORAMINA
ANTERIOR CRANIAL FOSSA
1. Cribriform plate: olfactory nerves
2. Foramen caecum: venous sinus (nasal sagittal sinus)
3. Anterior ethmoidal canal: anterior ethmoidal nerve and vessels
4. Posterior ethmoidal canal: posterior ethmoidal nerve and vessels

MIDDLE CRANIAL FOSSA

1. Optic canal
   a. optic nerve
   b. ophthalmic artery
2. Superior orbital fissure
   a. terminal branches of ophthalmic nerve
   b. 3rd, 4th and 6th cranial nerves
   c. meningeal branch of lacrimal artery
   d. ophthalmic veins
3. Foramen rotundum: maxillary nerve
4. Foramen ovale
   a. mandibular nerve
   b. accessory meningeal artery
   c. lesser superficial petrosal nerve
5. Foramen spinosum
   a. middle meningeal artery and veins
   b. nervus spinosus
6. Fossa lacerum
   a. internal carotid artery, sympathetic and venous plexi
   b. meningeal branches of accessory pharyngeal artery
   c. emissary veins
   d. greater superficial petrosal nerve joined by deep petrosal nerve to enter the pterygoid canal within the foramen
7. Hiatus for lesser petrosal nerve
8. Hiatus for greater petrosal nerve
9. Emissary sphenoidal foramen: emissary vein from cavernous sinus

POSTERIOR CRANIAL FOSSA

1. Foramen magnum
   a. medulla oblongata
   b. spinal roots of accessory nerve
   c. vertebral arteries with sympathetic plexus
   d anterior and posterior spinal arteries
2. Jugular foramen
   a. sigmoid sinus to internal jugular vein
   b. 9th, 10th and 11th cranial nerves
   c. inferior petrosal sinus
3. Within jugular foramen: openings of canals for:
   1. Aquaduct of cochlea
   2. Tympanic nerve branch of 9th nerve
   3. Auricular branch of 10th nerve
4. Hypoglossal canal
   1. XIIth nerve
   2. Meningeal branches of ascending pharyngeal artery

5. Internal acoustic meatus
   1. 7th and 8th nerves
   2. Internal auditory vessels
   3. Nervus intermedius
   4. Labyrinthine vessels
6. Mastoid foramen
   1. Emissary veins from sigmoid sinus
   2. Meningeal branch of occipital artery
7. Posterior condylar canal: emissary vein from sigmoid sinus
8. Facial canal: 7th nerve through petrous temporal bone to the stylomastoid foramen
9. Stylomastoid foramen
   1. Facial nerve
   2. Stylomastoid artery

OTHER OPENINGS IN THE SKULL
1. Supra-orbital foramen (frontal bone): supra-orbital vessels and nerves
2. Infra-orbital foramen (maxilla): infra-orbital vessels and nerves
3. Zygomaticofacial foramen (zygoma): zygomaticofacial nerve and artery
4. Zygomaticotemporal foramen (zygoma): zygomaticotemporal nerve and artery
5. Inferior orbital fissure (Sphenoid: inferior wall of orbit)
   a. maxillary nerve i.e.
   b. veins from ophthalmic to pterygoid plexus
   c. infra-orbital vessels
   d. zygomatic nerve
6. Nasolacrimal canal (lacrimal bone): nasolacrimal duct
7. Pterygomaxillary fissure
   a. terminal part maxillary artery
   b. maxillary nerve
8. Palatinovaginal canal: pharyngeal nerve and artery from pterygopalatine ganglion to roof of pharynx
9. Sphenopalatine foramen (palatine bone): nasopalatine (long sphenopalatine) nerve and artery
10. Greater palatine canal: anterior, middle and posterior palatine nerves. Greater and lesser palatine vessels
11. Greater palatine foramen (maxilla): greater (anterior) palatine nerve and vessels
12. Lesser palatine foramen (palatine bone): lesser (middle and posterior) palatine nerves and vessels
13. Mandibular foramen (mandible): inferior alveolar nerves and vessels
14. Mandibular canal (mandible): inferior alveolar nerves and vessels
15. Mental foramen (mandible): mental nerve and vessels

16. Petrotympanic fissure: anterior tympanic branch of maxillary artery. Chorda tympani
17. Incisive foramina
    a. termination of greater palatine vessels
    b. nasopalatine nerve
18. Parietal foramen (parietal bone): emissary vein from superior sagittal sinus

Orbit, ear and nose

ORBIT

The orbits are bilateral, pyramid-shaped concavities in the skull which contain the eyeball and extra-ocular structures.

POSITION
Roof
1. Orbital plate of frontal bone
2. Lesser wing of sphenoid bone

Medial wall
1. Anterior lacrimal crest of maxilla (anterior)
2. Lacrimal bone
3. Orbital plate of ethmoid bone
4. Body of sphenoid bone (posterior)

Lateral wall
1. Zygomatic bone
2. Greater wing of sphenoid bone

Floor
1. Orbital plate of maxilla (anterior)
2. Zygomatic bone
3. Orbital process of palatine bone (posterior)

EXTRA-OCULAR STRUCTURES

Extra-ocular
1. Eyelids and eyelashes
2. Orbicularis oculi
3. Lacrimal gland
4. Conjunctiva
5. Extra-ocular muscles
6. Vessels and nerves

Eyelids
1. Formed from
   a. loose skin (anterior)
   b. conjunctiva (posterior)
   c. tarsal plates (in between)
   d. palpebral part of orbicularis oculi
2. Blood supply: palpebral branch of ophthalmic artery

Orbicularis oculi
1. The facial muscle which surrounds the orbit
2. Nerve supply from zygomatic branch of facial nerve

Lacrimal gland
1. Position: superolateral margin of orbit
2. Ducts open into lateral part of the superior fornix of the conjunctiva
3. Nerve supply: secretomotor fibres from the superior salivatory nucleus via genicular ganglion, greater superficial petrosal nerve, pterygopalatine ganglion, zygomaticotemporal branch of maxillary nerve and then the lacrimal nerves

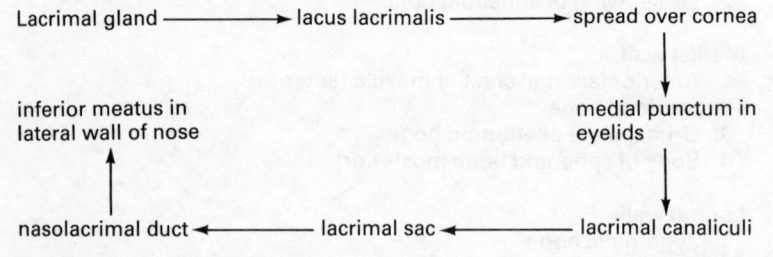

Lacrimal gland ⟶ lacus lacrimalis ⟶ spread over cornea
⟶ medial punctum in eyelids
⟶ lacrimal canaliculi ⟶ lacrimal sac ⟶ nasolacrimal duct ⟶ inferior meatus in lateral wall of nose

Fig. 28 Circulation of tears.

Conjunctiva
1. A transparent membrane
2. Stratified squamous epithelium (and columnar in parts)
3. Covers cornea
4. Covers internal surface of eyelids

Extra-ocular muscles
Many take origin from a fibrous ring which surrounds the optic foramen and the inferior part of the superior orbital fissure (see Table 3).

Table 3 Extraocular muscles

Name	Origin	Insertion	Nerve supply	Action on eyeball
Levator palpebrae superioris	Lesser wing of sphenoid	Superior tarsal plate Skin of upper eyelid	III	Elevate upper eyelid
Superior rectus	Fibrous ring	Superior part of eyeball	III	Elevation Adduction
Medial rectus	Fibrous ring	Medial part of eyeball	III	Adduction
Inferior rectus	Fibrous ring	Inferior part of eyeball Inferior tarsal plate	III	Adduction Depression Retraction of lower eyelid
Inferior oblique	Floor of anterior part of orbit	Postero inferior part of eyeball	III	Elevation Abduction
Lateral rectus	Fibrous ring	Lateral part of eyeball	VI	Abduction
Superior oblique	Above and medial to fibrous ring	Posterosuperior part of eyeball after passing through the trochlea on superomedial angle of orbital margin	IV	Depression Abduction

Vessels and nerves
These enter or leave the orbit via three main paths:
1. Superior orbital fissure
    a. lacrimal nerve
    b. frontal nerve
    c. trochlear nerve
    d. superior division of III
    e. nasociliary nerve
    f. inferior division of III
    g. abducent nerve
    h. superior ophthalmic vein
2. Optic foramen
    a. optic nerve
    b. ophthalmic artery

3. Inferior orbital fissure
   a. inferior ophthalmic vein
   b. infraorbital nerve
   c. zygomatic nerve

Lymph vessels drain the orbit to the pre-auricular and parotid lymph nodes.

INTRA-OCULAR STRUCTURES

Eyeball

The eyeball is surrounded by the fascia bulbi (Tenon's capsule) which attaches to the sclerocorneal junction and passes back to enclose the optic nerve.

Structure
1. Layers
   a. outer (sclera): which continues anteriorly as the cornea
   b. middle (vascular)
      (i) choroid
      (ii) ciliary body (and muscle)
      (iii) iris
   c. inner (retinal)
      (i) outer pigmented layer
      (ii) inner nervous layer
2. Lens
   a. connected to ciliary body by the suspensory ligament. Contraction of the ciliary muscle relaxes it, allowing the lens to accomodate
   b. separates the anterior segment of the eyeball (aqueous humour) from the posterior segment (vitreous humour)
3. Canal of Schlemm
   a. runs in sclerocorneal canal
   b. drains aqueous humour
4. Retina
   a. pigmented layer: nearest vitreous humour
   b. nervous layer: composed of rods and cones with their central connections
   c. optic disc: entrance of optic nerve
   d. macula lutea: posterior pole of retina
   e. fovea contralis: centre of macula
5. Iris
   a. attaches to the ciliary body anterior to the lens. It forms the pupil and contains the dilator and sphincter pupillae muscles
   b. it divides the anterior segment of the eyeball into anterior and posterior chambers

Blood supply
Ophthalmic artery
1. Anterior ciliary branches
2. Central artery of retina
3. Posterior ciliary branches
4. Branches which accompany lacrimal nerve, frontal nerve and nasociliary nerve

Nerve supply
1. Somatic: nasociliary nerve; sensory from cornea
2. Parasympathetic: inferior division of III
    a. sphincter pupillae
    b. ciliary muscle (accommodation)
3. Sympathetic: cavernous plexus to nasociliary nerve
    a. dilator pupillae
    b. vasoconstrictor to blood vessels of eye

EAR

The ear consists of three parts:
1. External ear
2. Middle ear
3. Inner ear

It has two main functions:
1. Hearing
2. Balance

EXTERNAL EAR

Structure
1. Pinna: yellow elastic cartilage covered with skin
2. External acoustic meatus
    a. 1 cm cartilage
    b. 2 cm bone (tympanic plate)
3. Tympanic membrane: separates external acoustic meatus from the middle ear

Nerve supply (sensory)
1. Auriculotemporal nerve
2. Lesser occipital nerve
3. Great auricular nerve
4. Auricular branch of Vagus nerve
5. Facial nerve

Motor fibres to small muscles acting on the pinna are supplied by the facial nerve.

Blood supply
1. Superficial temporal artery
2. Deep auricular branch of maxillary artery
3. Posterior auricular artery

MIDDLE EAR (TYMPANIC CAVITY)

The tympanic cavity is an air-filled cavity in the petrous part of the temporal bone.

Structures

Medial wall
1. Bony lateral wall of internal ear
2. Oval window (fenestra vestibuli)
   a. lateral: footpiece of stapes
   b. medial: perilymph of vestibule
3. Round window (fenestra cochlea): medial; perilymph of blind end of cochlea
4. Promontory: formed by prominence of part of cochlea and contains the nerves of the tympanic plexus
5. Prominence of the facial nerve canal

Lateral wall

  Tympanic membrane and epitympanic recess
1. Chorda tympani: crosses pars flaccida of tympanic membrane (posterior to anterior)
2. Tympanic membrane
   a. pars flaccida (superior)
   b. pars tensa (inferior)

Roof
Tegmen tympani (part of petrous bone)

Anterior wall
1. Auditory tube
2. Canal for tensor tympani
3. Branches of internal carotid artery

Floor
1. Tympanic plate (part of petrous bone)
2. Jugular fossa
3. Carotid canal
4. Jacobsen's nerve (tympanic branch of IX)

Posterior wall

  Mastoid antrum and aditus to mastoid antrum
Pyramidal eminence (contains stapedius)

Contents
Ossicles
1. Malleus
   a. head: articulates with incus
   b. neck
   c. handle
      (i) insertion of tensor tympani muscle
      (ii) connected to tympanic membrane
   d. anterior process: connected to petrotympanic fissure
   e. lateral process: connected to upper end of tympanic membrane
2. Incus
   a. body: articulates with head of malleus
   b. long process: articulates with head of stapes
   c. short process: connects to epitympanic recess
3. Stapes
   a. head: articulates with incus
   b. neck: insertion of stapedius muscle
   c. limbs: connect neck to base
   d. base: connects to the oval window

The articulations are synovial. The function of the ossicles is to connect the tympanic membrane to the inner ear, allowing transmission of sound waves

Muscles
1. Stapedius
   a. origin: pyramid on posterior wall
   b. insertion: neck of stapes
   c. nerve supply: facial nerve
   d. action: relaxes base of stapes in oval window, rendering the tympanic membrane less tense
2. Tensor Tympani
   a. origin: cartilaginous part of auditory tube
   b. insertion: handle of malleus
   c. nerve supply: branch of nerve to medial pterygoid (branch of mandibular branch of trigeminal nerve)
   d. action: draws tympanic membrane medially and presses base of stapes into oval window rendering the tympanic membrane more tense.

INNER EAR
The structures in the inner ear are too complex to be explained in detail here. Only the main parts and functions are summarized.

Bony labyrinth
This lies within the petrous part of the temporal bone, is lined with

periosteum and contains perilymph. It contains the membraneous labyrinth and consists of three parts.
1. Vestibule
2. Cochlea
3. Semi-circular canals

Vestibule
1. Lies between the cochlea (anterior) and the semi-circular canals (posterior)
2. Contains
   a. saccule
   b. utricle
   c. part of the endolymphatic duct

Cochlea
1. Conical in shape
2. The modiolus is the bone stem axis around which the cochlea spirals. It contains branches of the cochlear nerve. The spiral lamina is a shelf of bone projecting into the canal from the modiolus
3. It contains the Duct of cochlea
4. The basilar membrane divides the cochlea into two canals (scala tympani and scala vestibuli), which connect at the apex. It stretches from the modiolus to the outer wall in the cochlea
5. The vestibular membrane also runs from the modiolus to the outer wall of the cochlea. Between the vestibular and basilar membranes is the Organ of Corti

Semi-circular canals
1. Anterior (superior)
2. Posterior
3. Lateral
4. All at 90° to each other and 45° to sagittal plane
5. All form two-thirds of a circle
6. Dilated at one end to form the ampulla

The lateral canal opens at both ends into the vestibule while the ampulla of each of the anterior and posterior canals open separately into the vestibule; the other ends join to open as one canal into the vestibule.

Membraneous labyrinth
This is a continuous, closed cavity containing endolymph, which occupies the bony labyrinth.

Functions
1. Duct of cochlea: hearing
2. Saccule and utricle: static balance
3. Semicircular ducts: kinetic balance

The endolymphatic duct connects the utricle and saccule.

PATHWAYS OF HEARING AND BALANCE
See Figure 29.

Pathways of Hearing and Balance

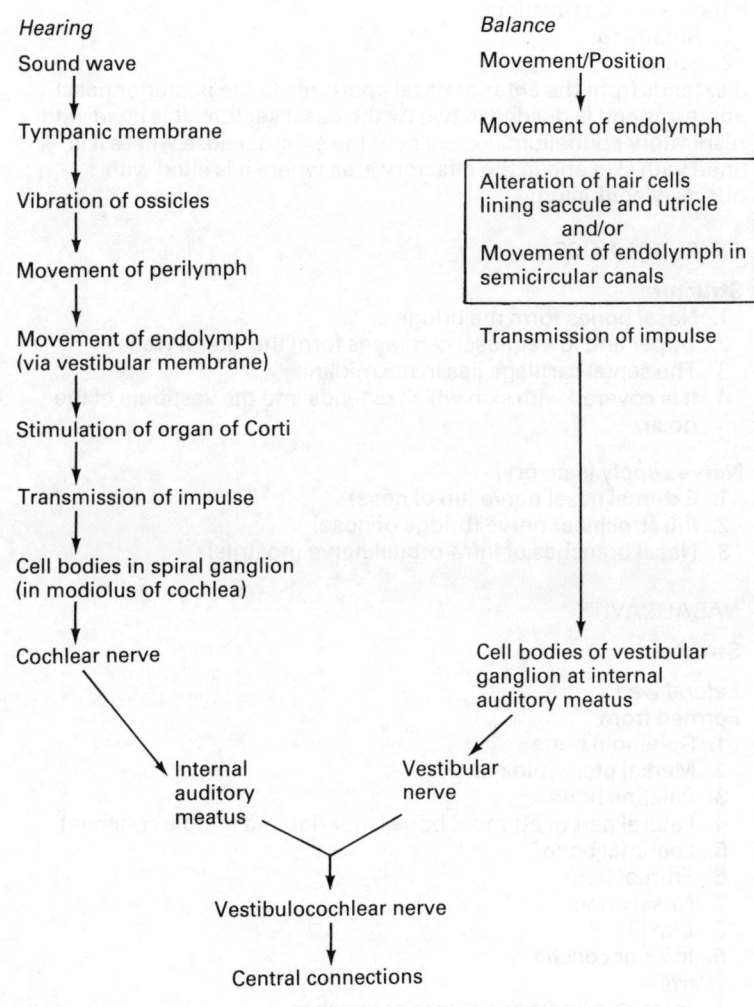

Hearing
Sound wave
↓
Tympanic membrane
↓
Vibration of ossicles
↓
Movement of perilymph
↓
Movement of endolymph
(via vestibular membrane)
↓
Stimulation of organ of Corti
↓
Transmission of impulse
↓
Cell bodies in spiral ganglion
(in modiolus of cochlea)
↓
Cochlear nerve
↓
Internal auditory meatus

Balance
Movement/Position
↓
Movement of endolymph
↓
> Alteration of hair cells
> lining saccule and utricle
> and/or
> Movement of endolymph in
> semicircular canals

↓
Transmission of impulse
↓
Cell bodies of vestibular
ganglion at internal
auditory meatus
↓
Vestibular nerve

↓
Vestibulocochlear nerve
↓
Central connections

Fig. 29 Pathways of hearing and balance.

NOSE

The nose comprises two parts:
1. External nose
2. Nasal cavity

It has two main functions:
1. Breathing
2. Smell

It extends from the anterior nasal apertures to the posterior nasal apertures and is divided in two by the nasal septum. It is lined with respiratory epithelium, except near the external nose where it is lined with skin and in the olfactory area where it is lined with olfactory epithelium.

EXTERNAL NOSE

Structure
1. Nasal bones form the bridge
2. Upper and lower nasal cartilages form the lateral walls
3. The septal cartilage lies in the midline.
4. It is covered with skin which extends into the vestibule of the nose

Nerve supply (sensory)
1. External nasal nerve (tip of nose)
2. Infratrochlear nerve (bridge of nose)
3. Nasal branches of infra-orbital nerve (nostrils)

NASAL CAVITY

Structure

Lateral wall
Formed from
1. Sphenoid bone
2. Medial pterygoid plate
3. Palatine bone
4. Lateral part of ethmoid bone (superior and middle conchae)
5. Lacrimal bone
6. Frontal bone
7. Nasal bone
8. Maxilla
9. Inferior concha.

Parts
1. Inferior, Middle and Superior conchae
2. Inferior meatus: lower orifice of nasolacrimal duct
3. Middle meatus
    a. ethmoidal bulla (ethmoidal air cells)
    b. uncinate process of ethmoid
    c. hiatus semiluminaris contains ostia of:

    (i) frontal sinus
    (ii) anterior ethmoidal sinuses
    (iii) middle ethmoidal sinuses
    (iv) ostium of maxillary sinus
4. Superior meatus: ostium of posterior ethmoidal air cells
5. Sphenopalatine foramen: opens posteriorly into the superior meatus
6. Spheno-ethmoidal recess
    a. Above superior concha
    b. Ostium of sphenoid air cells
    c. Sphenoidal sinus

Medial wall
1. Perpendicular plate of ethmoid bone
2. Vomer
3. Nasal cartilage

Posterior nasal apertures
1. Below: posterior border of horizontal plate of palatine bone
2. Above: base of skull
3. Lateral: medial pterygoid plate
4. Medial: vomer

Floor
1. Maxilla
2. Palatine bone (horizontal plate)

Roof
1. Nasal spine of nasal bone (anterior)
2. Nasal spine of frontal bone
3. Cribiform plate of ethmoid bone
4. Body of sphenoid (posterior)

Nerve and blood supply, venous and lymphatic drainage of nasal cavity

Lateral wall
1. Anterior superior quadrant
    a. anterior ethmoidal nerve
    b. anterior ethmoidal artery
    c. anterior facial vein
    d. submandibular lymph nodes
2. Anterior inferior quadrant
    a. submandibular lymph nodes
    b. anterior superior alveolar nerve
    c. anterior superior alveolar artery
    d. facial vein

3. Posterior superior quadrant
   a. posterior superior lateral nasal nerve
   b. posterior superior lateral nasal artery
   c. pharyngeal venus plexus
   d. deep cervical lymph nodes (retropharyngeal lymph nodes)
4. Posterior inferior quadrant
   a. pharyngeal venous plexus
   b. pterygoid venous plexus
   c. greater palatine nerve
   d. greater palatine artery
   e. deep cervical lymph nodes (retropharyngeal lymph nodes)

Medial wall
1. Anterior half
   a. facial artery
   b. anterior ethmoidal artery
   c. anterior ethmoidal nerve
   d. submandibular lymph nodes
   e. facial veins
2. Posterior half
   a. long sphenopalatine artery
   b. nasopalatine nerve
   c. retropharyngeal lymph nodes
   d. deep cervical lymph nodes
   e. pterygoid venous plexus

PARANASAL AIR SINUSES

These are all bilateral, air-filled cavities, lined with respiratory epithelium, which communicate with the nasal cavity and produce mucus.

Maxillary sinus (Antrum of Highmore)
1. Within maxilla
2. Lateral to nasal cavities
3. Inferior to orbits
4. Superior to the upper teeth

Ethmoidal sinus
1. Between orbit and nasal cavity
2. Within the lateral mass of ethmoid bone
3. Below orbital plate of ethmoid bone

Sphenoidal sinus
1. Within body of sphenoid bone
2. Beneath pituitary fossa

Frontal sinus
Within frontal bone

Fossae, triangles and canals

FOSSAE

PTERYGOPALATINE FOSSA

Roof
Body of sphenoid and orbital process of palatine bone communicates with orbit via inferior orbital fissure

Posterior wall
Pterygoid process of the greater wing of sphenoid

Medial wall
Perpendicular plate of palatine bone

Lateral wall
Communicates with infra-temporal fossa via pterygomaxillary fissure.

Anterior
Posterior surface of maxilla

Floor
Anterior and posterior walls come together

Contents
1. Maxillary nerve
2. Terminal part maxillary artery
3. Pterygo-palatine ganglion

Openings from and into the fossa

Roof
Inferior orbital fissure: maxillary nerve (out)

Posterior wall
1. Foramen rotundum: maxillary nerve (in)
2. Pterygoid canal: pterygoid nerve and artery (in)
3. Palatinovaginal canal: pharyngeal nerve and artery (out)

Medial wall
Sphenopalatine foramen
1. Nasopalatine nerve and artery (out)
2. Posterior superior lateral nasal nerves (out)

Inferior wall
Greater palatine canal
1. Anterior middle and posterior palatine nerves (out)
2. Greater and lesser palatine vessels (out)

Lateral wall
Pterygomaxillary fissure
1. Maxillary artery (in)
2. Posterior superior alveolar nerves (out)
3. Veins (out)

INFRATEMPORAL FOSSA

The infratemporal fossa lies behind maxilla, communicates with the orbit via the infra-orbital fissure, the pterygopalatine fossa via pterygomaxillary fissure, and the temporal fossa beneath the zygomatic arch.

Roof
Infratemporal surface of greater wing of sphenoid and part of the squamous temporal bone; roof pierced by foramen ovale and foramen spinosum

Medial wall
Lateral pterygoid plate completed in front and below by tubercle of palatine bone

Anterior wall
Posterior wall of maxilla

Posterior wall
Styloid apparatus and carotid sheath
Fossa open inferiorly and laterally

Contents
1. Maxillary artery and branches
2. Pterygoid venous plexus amongst lateral pterygoid muscle
3. Lateral and medial pterygoid muscle
4. Mandibular nerve enters via foramen ovale and breaks up into its branches in the fossa.
5. Chorda tympani

The maxillary nerve appears as it proceeds from pterygoid-maxillary fissure to the inferior orbital fissure.

The anterior wall is pierced by posterior superior alveolar vessels and nerves.

CUBITAL FOSSA

Triangular shape

Base
Line between humeral epicondyles

Medial side
Pronator teres

Lateral side
Brachioradialis

Floor
Brachialis, supinator

Roof
Skin, superficial fascia and reinforced by bicipital aponeurosis medially

Contents (medial to lateral)
1. Median nerve
2. Brachial artery and veins dividing into radial and ulnar branches
3. Tendon of biceps
4. Posterior interosseous nerve
5. Radial nerve

POPLITEAL FOSSA

Diamond shape

Lateral sides
1. Proximal: biceps femoris
2. Distal: Lateral head of gastrocnemius and plantaris

Medial sides
1. Proximal: semi-tendinosis and semi-membranosus
2. Distal: medial head gastrocnemius

Floor (from above down)
1. Popliteal surface of femur
2. Oblique posterior ligament of knee
3. Fascia overlying popliteus

Roof
Popliteal fascia and skin

Contents
1. Popliteal vessels
2. Tibial and common peroneal nerves
3. Termination of short saphenous vein
4. Lymph nodes
5. Articular branch of obturator nerve
6. Fat

AXILLA

Pyramidal region. Transmits vessels and nerves from the neck to arm.

Blunt apex
1. Towards root of the neck
2. Transmits the axillary vessels and nerves
3. Lies between the outer border of 1st rib, superior border of scapula and the posterior border of the clavicle

Base
Directed downwards. Formed by the skin and axillary fascia between pectoralis major in front and latissimus dorsi behind. Wider medially (against chest wall)

Anterior wall
1. Pectoralis major
2. Pectoralis minor
3. Clavipectoral fascia

Posterior wall
1. Subscapularis
2. Teres major
3. Latissimus dorsi

Medial wall
1. 1st four ribs and corresponding muscles
2. Serratus anterior

Lateral wall
1. Narrow as anterior and posterior walls converge
2. Bicipital groove of humerus
3. Coracobrachialis and biceps

Contents
1. Axillary artery and its branches
2. Axillary vein and tributaries
3. Infraclavicular part of brachial plexus and branches particularly nerve to subscapularis

4. Nerve to serratus anterior (long thoracic nerve of Bell)
  5. Thoracodorsal nerve
  6. Lateral branches of intercostal nerves
  7. Fat
  8. Lymph nodes: five groups
     a. pectoral
     b. subscapular
     c. lateral
     d. central
     e. apical

ISCHIORECTAL FOSSA

The ischiorectal fossae are wedge-shaped, one either side of rectum and anal canal and extend into urogenital triangle.

Base
Towards perineum

Apex
Formed by junction of obturator internus and levator ani

Medial
Two fossae separated by perineal body, anal canal and anococcygeal body

Lateral
  1. Ischial tuberosity
  2. Obturator fascia over obturator internus

Posterior
  1. Gluteus maximus
  2. Sacrotuberous ligament

Roof
Sloping fibres of levator ani

Anteriorly
  1. Extends as far as the posterior border of the urogenital diaphragm, with a recess extending forwards above urogenital diaphragm to posterior border of pubis
  2. Separated in the midline by membranous urethra and sphincter urethrae

Contents
  1. Inferior rectal vessels and nerve
  2. Perineal branch of S4

3. Perforating cutaneous branches of sacral plexus
4. Posterior scrotal/labial vessels and nerves
5. Pudendal canal is a condensation of fascia on the lateral wall of the fossa containing the internal pudendal vessels and nerve
6. Adipose tissue

TRIANGLES

ANTERIOR TRIANGLE OF THE NECK

Borders
1. Anterior: midline of the neck
2. Posterior: anterior border of sternomastoid
3. Base: inferior border of mandible and line from angle to mastoid process
4. Apex: sternum

The anterior triangle is divided into four.

Muscular triangle

Sides
1. Midline of neck; hyoid to sternum
2. Superior belly of omohyoid
3. Anterior border sternomastoid

Carotid triangle

Sides
1. Sternomastoid
2. Superior belly omohyoid
3. Stylohyoid and posterior belly digastric

Roof
Skin, fascia, platysma and deep fascia with branches of cutaneous nerves

Floor
Thyrohyoid, hyoglossus, inferior and middle constrictors

Contents
1. Common carotid artery and division into external and internal carotids
2. Branches of external carotid artery
   a. superior thyroid
   b. lingual
   c. occipital
   d. ascending pharyngeal with corresponding veins
3. Hypoglossal nerve giving off ansa cervicalis
4. Internal and external laryngeal nerves

Internal jugular vein and vagus lie *outside* the triangle, under the sternomastoid.

Digastric triangle

Sides
1. Inferior border of mandible and line from angle to mastoid process
2. Posterior belly of digastric and stylohyoid
3. Anterior belly digastric

Roof
Skin, fascia, platysma, deep fascia with cutaneous nerves

Floor
Mylohyoid, hyoglossus

Contents
1. Submandibular gland
2. Facial vessels
3. Submental artery
4. Mylohyoid vessels
5. Lower pole of parotid gland
6. External carotid artery
7. Internal carotid artery separated from external carotid by styloglossus, stylopharyngeus and glossopharyngeal nerve
8. Internal jugular vein
9. Vagus nerve

Submental triangle
1. Sides: anterior belly of digastric either side of midline
2. Base: hyoid bone
3. Floor: mylohyoid
4. Apex: mandible

Contents
1. Lymph nodes
2. Anterior jugular vein

POSTERIOR TRIANGLE OF NECK

Borders
1. Anterior: Sternomastoid
2. Posterior: Anterior border of trapezius
3. Base: Middle one-third of clavicle
4. Apex: Occipital bone between sternomastoid and trapezius

The posterior triangle is divided into two by inferior belly of omohyoid.

Occipital triangle

Sides
Sternomastoid and trapezius

Base
Inferior belly of omohyoid

Floor
Splenius capitis, levator scapulae, scalenus medius and posterior

Roof
Skin, fascia, platysma

Contents
1. Accessory nerve
2. Cervical plexus
3. Upper part brachial plexus
4. Chain of lymph nodes
5. Supraclavicular nerves
6. Transverse cervical vessels

Supraclavicular triangle

Sides
1. Inferior belly omohyoid
2. Middle one-third of clavicle

Base
Posterior border sternomastoid

Floor
1. 1st rib
2. Scalenus medius
3. Serratus anterior first digitation

Roof
Skin, fascia, platysma

Contents
1. Supraclavicular nodes
2. Third part of subclavian artery
3. Subclavian vein
4. Brachial plexus
5. Nerve to subclavius
6. External jugular vein entering subclavian vein
7. Lymph nodes

FEMORAL TRIANGLE

Sides
1. Medial edge of sartorius
2. Medial edge of adductor longus

Base
Inguinal ligament

Floor
1. Iliacus, psoas major,
2. Pectineus, adductor longus

Contents
1. Femoral artery and vein
2. Femoral nerve and branches
3. Fat, lymph nodes

LUMBAR TRIANGLE

Base
Iliac crest

Sides
1. Lateral edge of latissimus dorsi
2. Posterior edge of external oblique

TRIANGLE OF AUSCULTATION

Sides
1. Trapezius
2. Latissimus dorsi
3. Medial border of scapula

SUBOCCIPITAL TRIANGLE

Sides
1. Rectus capitis posterior major: above and medially
2. Obliquus capitis superior: above and laterally
3. Obliquus capitis inferior: below and laterally

Floor
1. Posterior atlanto-occipital membrane
2. Posterior arch of atlas

Roof
1. Semi-spinalis capitis
2. Longissimus capitis

Contents
1. Vertebral artery
2. Dorsal ramus of 1st cervical nerve

CANALS

ADDUCTOR (SUBSARTOTIAL) CANAL

Begins at the apex of the femoral triangle and ends at the adductor hiatus. Triangular in cross-section.

Sides
1. Vastus medialis
2. Adductor longus
3. Adductor magnus

Roof
1. Aponeurosis lying across the vessels
2. Sartorius lies on this aponeurosis

Contents
1. Femoral artery and vein
2. Saphenous nerve

INGUINAL CANAL

Oblique canal 4 cm long, slanting down and medially. It begins at the deep inguinal ring, marked medially by inferior epigastric vessels and ends at superficial inguinal ring, a hiatus in the external oblique aponeurosis marked by the pubic tubercle.

Anterior wall
Skin, superficial fascia and aponeurosis of external oblique. Lateral one-third is reinforced by internal oblique.

Posterior wall
Conjoint tendon, transversalis fascia and reflected inguinal ligament

Roof
Arched fibres of internal oblique and transversus abdominis

Floor
Inguinal ligament and medially the lacunar ligament

Contents
1. Spermatic cord: male
2. Round ligament: female
3. Ilio-inguinal: nerve; both

Endocrine glands

The endocrine glands are ductless and their secretions (hormones) are released directly into the circulation. The hormones act on distal target organs. Certain organs are discrete endocrine glands and, certain organs have endocrine cells within them, such as the islets of Langerhans in the pancreas. They form part of the complex homeostatic mechanisms necessary for survival of a large multicellular organism.

THE PITUITARY GLAND (HYPOPHYSIS CEREBRA)

The pituitary gland is ovoid in shape, has dimensions 12 × 8 mm and is 500 mg in weight. It runs continuous with the infundibulum (hypophysial stalk).

POSITION

It lies in the hypophyseal fossa of the sphenoid bone and is overlapped by a layer of dura mater (Diaphragma Sellae) which is penetrated by the infundibulum.

STRUCTURE

The gland is divided into two functional halves which include the infundibulum, and the median eminence (part of the hypothalamus).

Macroscopic

Neurohypophysis
Consists of:
 1. Median eminence
 2. Infundibular stem (cone of the infundibulum)
 3. Pars posterior of pituitary (neural lobe)

Adenohypophysis
Consists of:
1. Pars tuberalis
2. Pars anterior
3. Pars intermedia

Microscopic

Adenohypophysis: cell types
1. Pars anterior
   a. acidophils
      (i) somatotrophs: secrete growth hormone
      (ii) mammotrophs: secrete prolactin
      (iii) corticotrophs: secrete adrenocorticotrophic hormone (ACTH)
   b. basophils
      (i) thyrotrophs: secrete thyroid-stimulating hormone (TSH)
      (ii) gonadotrophs: secrete luteinizing hormone (LH) and follicle-stimulating hormone (FSH)
   c. chromophobes: non-secretory phase of all cell types
2. Pars intermedia: numerous B-cells containing α and β endorphins.
3. Pars tuberalis: undifferentiated cells with few α and β types

Cells are arranged in cords, columns and follicles of differing sizes. The pituitary is a highly vascular structure surrounded by thin-walled venous sinusoids.

Neurohypophysis
Consists of
1. The terminal ends of axons have originated from cell bodies in the hypothalamus (supra-optic and paraventricular nuclei). The cell bodies synthesise hormones which pass down the axons to the endings in the neurohypophysis where they are released.
   Hormones: Anti-diuretic hormone (ADH)
   Oxytocin
2. Pituicytes; dendritic cells within pars posterior. Non-excitable cells.

Multiple vascular sinusoids lie adjacent to the nerve endings.

ARTERIAL SUPPLY

There are superior and inferior hypophyseal arteries on both sides (branches of the internal carotid). They supply the neurohypophysis and form the superior capillary bed of the portal system. The adenohypophysis has virtually no arterial supply.

Endocrine glands

VENOUS SYSTEM

Portal system
This carries hormone-releasing factors between the hypothalamus and the adenohypophysis.

A superior capillary bed lies in the hypothalamus and drains into venous channels that run into the pars anterior and terminate in the inferior capillary bed.

Systemic drainage
The inferior hypophyseal veins drain the adenohypophysis and neurohypophysis into surrounding dural venous sinuses.

There are also complex systems of venous drainage that allow the secretions of the adeno- and neurohypophyses to form short feedback loops controlling the secretion of the various releasing factors and the hormones.

THYROID GLAND

This is a brownish-red organ lying in the neck secreting thyroid hormones which are involved in the control of numerous metabolic pathways. It also has a role in calcium homeostasis. It weighs 25g.

POSITION
Anterior part of the neck at the level of C5 6 7 T1. It is enclosed in a pretracheal layer of deep cervical fascia.

STRUCTURE

Macroscopic
1. Right and left lobes with upper and lower poles
2. Connected across the midline by the isthmus. Occasionally a pyramidal pole is present

Microscopic
1. Capsule of connective tissue which divides glands into follicles
2. Two types of secretory cell:
   a. follicular: secrete tri-iodothyronin T_3 and thyroxine T_4.
   b. parafollicular (C-cells): secrete calcitonin
3. Form follicles 0.02–0.9 mm across which contain colloid. Size of follicle and amount of colloid depend on the secretory state of the gland

ARTERIAL SUPPLY

1. Superior thyroid artery: branch of external carotid
2. Inferior thyroid artery: branch of thyrocervical trunk
3. Arteria thyroidae ima: direct from aortic arch

VENOUS DRAINAGE

1. Superior thyroid vein ⎫
2. Middle thyroid vein   ⎬ to internal jugular vein
3. Inferior thyroid vein to left brachiocephalic vein

LYMPHATIC DRAINAGE

Groups of nodes in the neck and mediastinum
1. Prelaryngeal
2. Pretracheal
3. Paratracheal
4. Deep cervical
5. Brachiocephalic

NERVE SUPPLY

Sympathetic from superior, middle and inferior cervical ganglia.

PARATHYROID GLANDS

There are four parathyroid glands. They are yellowish brown ovoid glands, $6 \times 4 \times 2$ mm with each weighing 50 mg each. There are two on either side, superior and inferior. Inferior parathyroids develop from the third and the superior from the fourth pharyngeal pouches. They are involved in control of calcium metabolism.

POSITION

1. Superior gland: behind posterior border of upper part of thyroid within the capsule
2. Inferior gland: position is variable:
   1. Within thyroid fascia below inferior thyroid artery
   2. Outside thyroid fascia above inferior thyroid artery
   3. Within the substance of the thyroid

STRUCTURE

Thin capsule and fibrous septa divide each gland into lobular form

CELL TYPES

1. Principal/chief cells: secrete parathormone (PTH)
2. Oxyphil (eosinophils): unknown function

Cells arranged in columns surrounded by rich venous sinusoidal network.

Endocrine glands

ARTERIAL SUPPLY
1. Inferior thyroid artery
2. Anastomotic artery between superior and inferior thyroid arteries

VENOUS DRAINAGE
Corresponding veins

LYMPHATIC DRAINAGE
1. With LD of thyroid and thymus
2. Tracheal plexus ⎫
3. Prelaryngeal nodes ⎪
4. Pretracheal nodes ⎬ within the neck
5. Paratracheal nodes ⎪
6. Deep cervical nodes ⎭
7. Brachiocephalic nodes ⎫
8. Tracheobronchial nodes ⎬ in mediastinum
9. Parasternal nodes ⎭

NERVE SUPPLY
Sympathetic: via middle or superior cervical ganglia.

SUPRARENAL GLANDS
Two yellowish bodies, situated either side of midline. The suprarenal glands are made up of two separate functional parts: the cortex and the medulla. Their dimensions are 50 × 30 × 10 mm and weigh 5 mg.

POSITION
Retroperitoneal. They sit atop the kidneys within renal fascia.
1. Right gland: pyramidal — 'Cocked Hat'
2. Left gland: semilunar — larger than right gland

STRUCTURE
Macroscopic
1. Cortex: nine-tenths of gland — yellow colour
2. Medulla: one-tenth of gland — dark red. Enclosed by cortex except at hilum

Thick, fibrous capsule with rich plexus of arteries — Divide gland with fibrous septa.

Microscopic
1. Cortex (three zones)
    a. outer: zona glomerulosa cells produce aldosterone
    b. middle: zona fasciculata cells produce cortisol
    c. inner: zona reticularis cells produce sex hormones
2. Medulla: columns of chromaffin cells (phaeochromatocytes) produce adrenaline and noradrenaline. Wide venous sinusoids lie amongst the columns

ARTERIAL SUPPLY

1. Inferior phrenic artery: superior suprarenal artery
2. Aorta: middle suprarenal artery
3. Renal artery: inferior suprarenal artery

VENOUS DRAINAGE

Suprarenal vein to a. IVC on the right
                         b. Left renal vein on the left

LYMPHATIC DRAINAGE

Direct to lateral aortic nodes

NERVE SUPPLY

To medulla: pre-ganglionic sympathetic nerves from the greater splanchnic nerve

PINEAL GLAND

8 mm in length, the pineal gland is a reddish-grey organ occupying the space between the superior colliculi. It is an endocrine gland which modulates the activity of the adenohypophysis, neurohypophysis, endocrine pancreas, parathyroid, adrenal cortex and medulla, and the gonads.

Secretions are in general inhibitory. It secretes melatonins which show a circadian rhythm in man related to darkness and light.

STRUCTURE

1. Pinealocytes
2. Neuroglial cells: arranged in cords and follicles which lie amongst numerous blood vessels and nerve fibres, which are non-myelinated noradrenergic type.

CAROTID BODIES

The carotid bodies are two reddish-brown elliptical structures which function as arterial chemoreceptors.

POSITION

6 × 4 mm in size, the carotid bodies are situated on either side of the neck close to the carotid sinus. They lie at the bifurcation of the common carotid artery attached to its outer layers.

STRUCTURE

1. Capsulated organ divided into lobules
2. Collections of
   a. type 1 (glomus) cells
   b. type 2 (sheath) cells
3. Cells lie amongst venous sinusoids and numerous non-myelinated nerve fibres

ARTERIAL SUPPLY

From the branches of the external carotid artery.

VENOUS DRAINAGE

Corresponding vein

NERVE SUPPLY

Glossopharyngeal nerve. Components from vagus and sympathetic nerves join it to form a fine nerve plexus.

Skin and breast

SKIN

The skin is a specialized boundary which completely covers the body, being continuous with mucosal surfaces at each orifice. It is the major interface between the body and the environment. It protects the body from physical injury, attack by microorganisms and acts as a heat regulator. It also has a role in the synthesis of vitamin D. It is a social communicator with vascular responses and muscular expressions, and is a major sensory organ.

Two types of skin
1. Thin hairy skin: hairs, sebaceous glands. Covers the majority of the body
2. Thick glabrous skin: no hairs or sebaceous glands, e.g. Palms of hands and soles of feet

Pigmentation of skin
1. Results from
   a. melanin
   b. melanoid
   c. carotene
2. Final colour of the skin is also affected by vascularity

STRUCTURE

1. Two layers
   a. dermis (corum): connective tissue layer. Develops from mesenchyme
   b. epidermis: epithelium. Develops from ectoderm
2. Interface between the two layers arranged as
   a. peg and socket
   b. ridge and groove

Epidermis
1. Mechanical barrier
2. Regenerates itself
3. Forms the skin appendages
4. Has *no* direct blood supply

Types of surface marking
1. Tension lines: resulting in polygonal-shaped areas. See dorsum of hand
2. Flexure lines: correspond to joint movements
3. Papillary ridges
   a. palmar surface of hand and soles of feet
   b. forms the fingerprint

Microscopic
1. Keratinising stratified squamous epithelium
2. Varying thickness of keratin, depending on situation

The epidermis has two zones comprised of five layers.
1. Germinative zone
   a. stratum basale (basal cell layer: deepest layer)
   b. stratum spinosum (prickle cell layer)
      Other cell types within the germinative zone are:
         (i) melanocytes: synthesize melanin
         (ii) langerhans cell: macrophage of the skin
         (iii) merkel cell: involved in sensation
2. Zone of keratinisation
   a. stratum granulosum
   b. stratum lucidum
   c. stratum corneum (outer layer)

Dermis
This gives mechanical strength to skin. It is thick on palms of hands soles of feet but thin on the eyelids and scrotum

Microscopic
The dermis comprises two layers
1. Reticular layer (deep)
   a. fibrous and elastic tissue, formed into parallel bundles
   b. give rise to the cleavage lines
   c. contains fat and sweat glands between the bundles
2. Papillary layer (superficial): consists of conical projections of a sensitive and vascular nature known as papillae which interdigitate with the epidermis

VASCULAR SUPPLY AND DRAINAGE OF SKIN
Supply
1. Arteries penetrate the superficial fascia to form a plexus at the interface with the dermis: the rete cutaneum
2. Superficial plexus at the junction of the reticular papillary layers in the dermis reticular papillary layers: the rete subpapillare
3. Capillary loops run into each papilla

Drainage
From capillary beds to three venous plexus
1. Beneath the rete subpapillare
2. Within reticular layer of the dermis
3. Deep laminar plexus at the junction of dermis and superficial fascia

Multiple arteriovenous anastomoses in the dermis allow heat regulation

LYMPHATIC DRAINAGE
Networks
1. In papillary layer
2. In reticular layer of the dermis
3. Junction of dermis and superficial fascia

INNERVATION
Somatic sensory
1. Myelinated
2. Non-myelinated

Specialized sensory nerve endings
1. Merkels disc
2. Meissners corpuscle
3. Pacinian corpuscle
4. Bulbous corpuscle (of Krause)

Autonomic
Non-myelinated
1. Blood vessels
2. Pilomotor (smooth muscle)
3. Sweat glands

The nerve plexus in the papillary layer is called the dermal plexus.

SKIN APPENDAGES
Nail
1. Elastic horny structure
2. Grow 0.5 mm per week
3. Nail bed: germinal matrix

Hairs
1. Shaft
2. Root: the base of the root is the bulb where growth occurs
3. Follicle is invagination of epidermis; arrector pilae muscle fibres insert into base of follicle

Sebaceous glands
1. Holocrine glands which produce sebum cutaneum under hormonal control
2. Absent on palms of hands, soles and feet.

Sweat glands
Eccrine
1. Most numerous in axillae and groin
2. Merocrine in nature
3. Coiled single tubes
4. Concerned with temperature regulation

Apocrine
1. Thicker secretion
2. Occurs
   a. axillae
   b. eyelids
   c. areola and nipple
   d. circumaural
   e. external genitalia
3. Possible role in sexual attraction

Nerve supply
eccrine: Cholinergic sympathetic
apocrine: Dual autonomic supply

BREAST
Breast tissue is present in both the male and female, although it remains rudimentary in the male. It develops at puberty in the female, with the largest development occurring in pregnancy and after parturition; it provides milk for the newborn. Breast tissue, consists of glandular tissue, adipose tissue and fibrous tissue. It is described as an apocrine type gland.

POSITION
1. Lies in superficial fascia over the thoracic wall
2. Shape and consistency are individual

Base of the breast
The base is constant
1. Vertically 2nd–6th ribs
2. Transversely from sternum to mid axillary line
3. Axillary tail superolateral prolongation
4. Submammary space: loose areolar tissue beneath breast, superficial to deep fascia

Nipple
1. On anterior surface of breast
2. Level of 4th intercostal space
3. Pink/light brown colour
4. 15–20 lactiferous ducts open on its surface
5. Numerous smooth muscle fibres

Areola
1. Encircles the nipple
   a. pink: nulliparous
   b. brown: pregnancy
2. Numerous sebaceous glands: 'Montgomery's tubercles'

STRUCTURE

Macroscopic

Tissue components
1. Glandular tissue: 15–20 lobes
2. Fibrous tissue: connecting lobes and form suspensory ligaments of Cooper
3. Adipose tissue: between lobes

Lobes
1. Divided into lobules: each lobule consists of clusters of rounded alveoli
2. Drain into one lactiferous duct
3. Dilatation below nipple of each duct to form the lactiferous sinus

Microscopic

Alveoli
Lined by secretory-cuboidal/columnar epithelium

Ducts
Lined by columnar epithelium. Stratified squamous epithelium towards the opening on the nipple.

Myoepithelial cells
Beneath the lining cells of alveoli and ducts, they cause passage of milk, when stimulated by suckling reflex (oxytocin).

Changes
Structure varies with age, and pregnancy, under influence of hormonal environments.
1. Before puberty: lactiferous ducts; no alveoli
2. At puberty: ducts branch and form potential alveoli
3. Pregnancy
    a. Develop secretory alveoli which produce colostrum around time of birth
    b. True milk produced post-parturition, under the influence of prolactin

ARTERIAL SUPPLY

1. Axillary artery via
    a. lateral thoracic artery
    b. thoraco-acromial artery: pectoral branch
2. Internal thoracic (mammary) artery
    a. perforating branches
    b. anterior intercostal branches
3. Intercostal arteries: mammary branches

VENOUS DRAINAGE

1. Circulus venous around base of nipple
2. Drain to corresponding veins, of main arterial supply

LYMPHATIC DRAINAGE

1. Subareolar plexus
2. Axillary nodes
    a. pectoral group receive 75% of drainage
    b. subscapular group
    c. apical group
3. Parasternal nodes along internal thoracic artery
4. Few branches via anterior intercostal arteries to intercostal nodes

NERVE SUPPLY

1. Sensory, autonomic via anterior and lateral cutaneous branches of 4th, 5th and 6th intercostal nerves
2. Dense nerve plexus around nipple: important in suckling reflex